Chronic Rhinosinusitis and Concomitant Medical Disorders

Chronic Rhinosinusitis and Concomitant Medical Disorders

Special Issue Editor
David A. Gudis

MDPI • Basel • Beijing • Wuhan • Barcelona • Belgrade • Manchester • Tokyo • Cluj • Tianjin

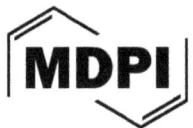

Special Issue Editor
David A. Gudis
Columbia University Irving
Medical Center, Department of
Otolaryngology-Head and
Neck Surgery
USA

Editorial Office
MDPI
St. Alban-Anlage 66
4052 Basel, Switzerland

This is a reprint of articles from the Special Issue published online in the open access journal *Medical Sciences* (ISSN 2076-3271) (available at: https://www.mdpi.com/journal/medsci/special_issues/Rhinosinusitis).

For citation purposes, cite each article independently as indicated on the article page online and as indicated below:

LastName, A.A.; LastName, B.B.; LastName, C.C. Article Title. *Journal Name* **Year**, *Article Number*, Page Range.

ISBN 978-3-03928-811-3 (Pbk)
ISBN 978-3-03928-812-0 (PDF)

© 2020 by the authors. Articles in this book are Open Access and distributed under the Creative Commons Attribution (CC BY) license, which allows users to download, copy and build upon published articles, as long as the author and publisher are properly credited, which ensures maximum dissemination and a wider impact of our publications.

The book as a whole is distributed by MDPI under the terms and conditions of the Creative Commons license CC BY-NC-ND.

Contents

About the Special Issue Editor vii

David A. Gudis
Introduction to "Chronic Rhinosinusitis and Concomitant Medical Disorders"
Reprinted from: *Med. Sci.* **2020**, *8*, 17, doi:10.3390/medsci8010017 1

Zhong Zheng, Chetan Safi and David A. Gudis
Surgical Management of Chronic Rhinosinusitis in Cystic Fibrosis
Reprinted from: *Med. Sci.* **2019**, *7*, 57, doi:10.3390/medsci7040057 3

Landon Massoth, Cody Anderson and Kibwei A. McKinney
Asthma and Chronic Rhinosinusitis: Diagnosis and Medical Management
Reprinted from: *Med. Sci.* **2019**, *7*, 53, doi:10.3390/medsci7040053 9

Kevin L. Li, Andrew Y. Lee and Waleed M. Abuzeid
Aspirin Exacerbated Respiratory Disease: Epidemiology, Pathophysiology, and Management
Reprinted from: *Med. Sci.* **2019**, *7*, 45, doi:10.3390/medsci7030045 25

Ryan Belcher and Frank Virgin
The Role of the Adenoids in Pediatric Chronic Rhinosinusitis
Reprinted from: *Med. Sci.* **2019**, *7*, 35, doi:10.3390/medsci7020035 43

Chetan Safi, Zhong Zheng, Emily Dimango, Claire Keating and David A. Gudis
Chronic Rhinosinusitis in Cystic Fibrosis: Diagnosis and Medical Management
Reprinted from: *Med. Sci.* **2019**, *7*, 32, doi:10.3390/medsci7020032 49

Sonya Marcus, John M. DelGaudio, Lauren T. Roland and Sarah K. Wise
Chronic Rhinosinusitis: Does Allergy Play a Role?
Reprinted from: *Med. Sci.* **2019**, *7*, 30, doi:10.3390/medsci7020030 57

Akira Kanda, Kenji Kondo, Naoki Hosaka, Yoshiki Kobayashi, Dan Van Bui, Yasutaka Yun, Kensuke Suzuki, Shunsuke Sawada, Mikiya Asako, Akihiko Nakamura, Koichi Tomoda, Yoshiko Sakata, Koji Tsuta, David Dombrowicz, Hideyuki Kawauchi, Shigeharu Fujieda and Hiroshi Iwai
Eosinophilic Upper Airway Inflammation in a Murine Model Using an Adoptive Transfer System Induces Hyposmia and Epithelial Layer Injury with Convex Lesions
Reprinted from: *Med. Sci.* **2019**, *7*, 22, doi:10.3390/medsci7020022 65

About the Special Issue Editor

David A. Gudis, M.D., is the Chief of the Division of Rhinology and Anterior Skull Base Surgery in the Department of Otolaryngology—Head and Neck Surgery at Columbia University Irving Medical Center/New York-Presbyterian Hospital. In addition to being a board-certified otolaryngologist, Dr. Gudis is dual-fellowship trained both in Rhinology: Advanced Endoscopic Sinus and Skull Base Surgery and in Pediatric Otolaryngology. Dr. Gudis was recruited to Columbia in 2015 and treats the full spectrum of sinonasal and skull base disorders in both adults and children. His practice includes the treatment of refractory and recurrent sinus disease, sinus and nasal tumors, minimally invasive endoscopic skull base surgery, and endoscopic orbital surgery. He collaborates closely with Neurosurgery, Oculoplastics Surgery, and Pulmonology in the care of complex patients.

Dr. Gudis pursued his medical education at the University of Pennsylvania Perelman School of Medicine, where he was the recipient of the Russel J. Stumacher M.D. Award. He then completed his residency in Otorhinolaryngology—Head and Neck Surgery at the University of Pennsylvania and the Children's Hospital of Philadelphia (CHOP). He completed a fellowship in Pediatric Otolaryngology and Craniofacial Surgery, followed by a fellowship in Rhinology: Advanced Endoscopic Sinus and Skull Base Surgery, at the Medical University of South Carolina in Charleston, South Carolina.

Dr. Gudis' clinical interests include the medical and surgical treatment of chronic sinusitis, revision sinus surgery, sinonasal polyposis, sinonasal tumors, skull base tumors, cerebrospinal fluid (CSF) leaks, endoscopic skull base surgery, and endoscopic orbital surgery. His research interests include rhinologic conditions in patients with pulmonary disease, such as cystic fibrosis and asthma, and novel surgical techniques for minimally invasive endoscopic skull base surgery for brain tumors and orbital tumors. He is the author of over 50 peer-reviewed publications and textbook chapters, and he is co-editor of a forthcoming textbook *The Unified Airway: Rhinologic Disease and Respiratory Disorders*. He is regularly invited to present his research at national and international conferences. He is on several national committees for rhinology, pediatric otolaryngology, and humanitarian efforts for national otolaryngology societies.

Dr. Gudis is passionate about health care and education for patients home and abroad. He is the Associate Director of the New York-Presbyterian/Cornell/Columbia Rhinology Fellowship, for advanced sinus and skull base surgery. He is also the Co-Director of the annual Columbia University Endoscopic Otolaryngology Course, which has trained otolaryngologists from over 15 different countries around the world in the latest techniques for advanced endoscopic sinus and skull base surgery. He is the recipient of several grants funding humanitarian missions to provide surgery, clinical care and research in underserved regions around the world, including in Haiti, Rwanda, Kenya, Ghana, the Dominican Republic, and Peru.

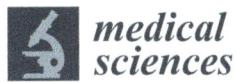

Editorial

Introduction to "Chronic Rhinosinusitis and Concomitant Medical Disorders"

David A. Gudis

Chief, Division of Rhinology & Anterior Skull Base Surgery; Department of Otolaryngology–Head and Neck Surgery, Columbia University Irving Medical Center, New York, NY 10032, USA; dag62@cumc.columbia.edu

Received: 16 March 2020; Accepted: 20 March 2020; Published: 23 March 2020

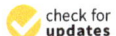

It is with great pleasure and enthusiasm that we present to you this Special Issue of Medical Sciences. In this issue, we present a comprehensive and contemporary review of the relationship between chronic rhinosinusitis and other respiratory disorders and, moreover, how our medical and surgical interventions as otolaryngologists impact those respiratory conditions. Our understanding of chronic rhinosinusitis has evolved tremendously over the last two decades. As we have learned, chronic rhinosinusitis—a chronic inflammatory condition of the nasal cavity and paranasal sinuses—is often a local inflammatory response to a systemic or mucosal disorder. The underlying systemic medical conditions not only influence the presentation and diagnosis of chronic rhinosinusitis, but also modify patients' responses to medical and surgical interventions. Chronic rhinosinusitis associated with cystic fibrosis, for example, is a disorder quite distinct from that associated with aspirin-exacerbated respiratory disease.

A clear understanding of the nuances that distinguish these unique and challenging disorders is critical for the practicing otolaryngologist. Equally important, however, is a clear understanding of the powerful benefits that our interventions as otolaryngologists can have for our patients' rhinologic and systemic health. Knowing that our rhinologic interventions might spare an asthma patient a trip to an emergency room, or reduce lung infections in a cystic fibrosis patient, makes this a very exciting time to be a rhinologist.

This compendium includes basic science, translational, and clinical evidence demonstrating the pathophysiology and treatment outcomes of inflammatory respiratory disorders. Dr. Kanda and colleagues examine the impact of eosinophilic inflammation, seen in clinical disorders such as asthma and aspirin-exacerbated respiratory disease, on airway epithelium in a murine model [1]. Dr. Safi et al. [2] and Dr. Zheng et al. [3] respectively explore the contemporary medical and surgical management paradigms of cystic fibrosis, in addition to treatment impact on pulmonary and systemic health. Dr. Massoth and colleagues [4] discuss the relationship between asthma and chronic rhinosinusitis, and Dr. Li and colleagues [5] further examine aspirin-exacerbated respiratory disease. Finally, Dr. Belcher et al. [6] and Dr. Marcus et al. [7] explore the common comorbidities of adenoiditis and allergic rhinitis, respectively, and how such concomitant disorders may impact the presentation, management, and outcomes of these patients.

We hope you enjoy this Special Issue of Medical Sciences.

Conflicts of Interest: The author declares no conflict of interest.

References

1. Kanda, A.; Kondo, K.; Hosaka, N.; Kobayashi, Y.; Bui, D.; Yun, Y.; Suzuki, K.; Sawada, S.; Asako, M.; Nakamura, A.; et al. Eosinophilic Upper Airway Inflammation in a Murine Model Using an Adoptive Transfer System Induces Hyposmia and Epithelial Layer Injury with Convex Lesions. *Med. Sci.* **2019**, *7*, 22. [CrossRef] [PubMed]

2. Safi, C.; Zheng, Z.; Dimango, E.; Keating, C.; Gudis, D. Chronic Rhinosinusitis in Cystic Fibrosis: Diagnosis and Medical Management. *Med. Sci.* **2019**, *7*, 32. [CrossRef] [PubMed]
3. Zheng, Z.; Safi, C.; Gudis, D. Surgical Management of Chronic Rhinosinusitis in Cystic Fibrosis. *Med. Sci.* **2019**, *7*, 57. [CrossRef] [PubMed]
4. Massoth, L.; Anderson, C.; McKinney, K. Asthma and Chronic Rhinosinusitis: Diagnosis and Medical Management. *Med. Sci.* **2019**, *7*, 53. [CrossRef] [PubMed]
5. Li, K.; Lee, A.; Abuzeid, W. Aspirin Exacerbated Respiratory Disease: Epidemiology, Pathophysiology, and Management. *Med. Sci.* **2019**, *7*, 45. [CrossRef]
6. Belcher, R.; Virgin, F. The Role of the Adenoids in Pediatric Chronic Rhinosinusitis. *Med. Sci.* **2019**, *7*, 35. [CrossRef]
7. Marcus, S.; DelGaudio, J.; Roland, L.; Wise, S. Chronic Rhinosinusitis: Does Allergy Play a Role? *Med. Sci.* **2019**, *7*, 30. [CrossRef] [PubMed]

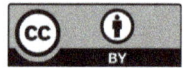

© 2020 by the author. Licensee MDPI, Basel, Switzerland. This article is an open access article distributed under the terms and conditions of the Creative Commons Attribution (CC BY) license (http://creativecommons.org/licenses/by/4.0/).

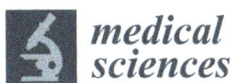

Review

Surgical Management of Chronic Rhinosinusitis in Cystic Fibrosis

Zhong Zheng, Chetan Safi and David A. Gudis *

Department of Otolaryngology—Head and Neck Surgery, Columbia University Irving Medical Center, New York, NY 10032, USA; zz2618@cumc.columbia.edu (Z.Z.); cys9028@nyp.org (C.S.)
* Correspondence: dag62@cumc.columbia.edu; Tel.: +1-212-305-8555

Received: 16 January 2019; Accepted: 5 April 2019; Published: 7 April 2019

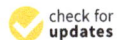

Abstract: Cystic fibrosis patients frequently develop chronic rhinosinusitis as a result of their propensity to form inspissated mucus and impairment of mucociliary clearance. They exhibit variable symptom burden even in the setting of positive radiographic and endoscopic findings. Current evidence suggests a positive effect of managing sinonasal disease on pulmonary health. Topical antimicrobial and mucolytic therapies are frequently required to manage the disease with surgery reserved for refractory cases. Endoscopic sinus surgery has been demonstrated to be safe and efficacious in controlling symptoms of chronic rhinosinusitis in patients with comorbid cystic fibrosis. However, the impact of surgery on pulmonary health remains an active area of investigation. In addition, a growing body of research has suggested a more extended surgical approach creating large sinonasal cavities with gravity-dependent drainage pathways, followed by adjuvant medical therapies, as an ideal strategy to optimally control disease and prevent pulmonary exacerbations. In this manuscript, we provide an up-to-date review of current evidence in the surgical management of chronic rhinosinusitis in cystic fibrosis patients.

Keywords: rhinosinusitis; cystic fibrosis; endoscopic sinus surgery; medial maxillectomy

1. Introduction

Cystic fibrosis (CF) is an autosomal recessive disease characterized by a defect in the cystic fibrosis transmembrane conductance regulator (CFTR) gene on chromosome 7, which encodes for a chloride ion transporter on the apical membrane of epithelial cells. It predominantly affects the Caucasian population, with a prevalence of ~30,000 patients in the United States and ~70,000 patients worldwide [1]. As a result of defective trans-membrane anion transport, CF patients develop increased epithelial sodium and water resorption and produce thick inspissated secretions, which then cause mucociliary stasis, chronic inflammation, bacterial colonization, and infection in multiple organ systems, including the upper and lower airways. The average life expectancy of CF patients is 48.5 years, and the majority of CF-related mortalities are due to progressive pulmonary decline, with many patients eventually requiring lung transplantation [2,3].

Impaired sinonasal mucociliary clearance mechanisms predispose CF patients to develop chronic rhinosinusitis (CRS) and nasal polyposis. On computed tomography (CT), CF patients also have under-developed paranasal sinuses due to chronic inflammation, further complicating ventilation and drainage [4]. Furthermore, a growing body of research has demonstrated a significant link between sinonasal and pulmonary health with regards to bacterial colonization, with an 80% concordance of bacterial isolates from sinonasal and bronchoalveolar lavages (BAL) [5]. The mainstays of medical therapies for CF CRS include oral and topical antibiotics directed at *Pseudomonas aeruginosa* and *Staphyloccocus aureus* species, topical mucolytic agents, and more recently CFTR modulators [6]. Refractory to medical therapy, endoscopic sinus surgery (ESS) has been shown to improve sinonasal symptoms and quality of life outcomes and reduce pulmonary bacterial colonization [5,7]. However, currently available data on the effect of ESS on pulmonary functions are conflicting [5,8]. In this manuscript, our objective is to provide an up-to-date review of current evidence in the surgical management of CRS in CF patients.

2. Unified Airway Health

Drawing a parallel with the unified airway model in reactive airway disease, mounting evidence has demonstrated a significant correlation between the health of paranasal sinuses and lungs. Studies have shown a possible mechanism of bacterial translocation from upper to lower airways. Therefore, in addition to alleviating symptoms of CRS in CF, ESS has the added benefit of creating an open and accessible sinonasal cavity to topical therapies and reducing bacterial seeding of the lungs. Furthermore, the reduction or eradication of pulmonary pathogenic colonization is critically important to prevent allograft rejection in post-lung transplant CF patients. A recent study compared microbiota composition from the sinuses and lung brushings using 16s RNA sequencing techniques, and microbiome diversity was found to be diminished in both the sinuses and lungs in CF CRS patients. Interestingly, non-CF CRS patients had distinct niches of microorganisms in their upper versus lower airways, while CF CRS patients had indistinguishable niches at both anatomic sites, lending further evidence to the theory of sinonasal cavity as a reservoir for bacterial translocation to lower airway in CF patients [9]. Walter and colleagues followed a cohort of 11 CF patients pre- and post-lung transplant, and identical *P. aeruginosa* isolates were seen in all patients within the sinuses and lungs [10]. Moreover, Mainz et al evaluated 182 CF patients and demonstrated significant genotypic concordance of *P. aeruginosa* and *S. aureus* isolates in upper and lower airways. Genetically identical strains of *P. aeruginosa* and *S. aureus* were identified in 31 of 36 and 23 of 24 patients, respectively. In addition, patients with positive *P. aeruginosa* sputum cultures were 88 times more likely to be colonized in the upper airway with the same bacterial pathogen [11]. In a different study, the same authors also found rapid colonization of new donor lungs with *P. aeruginosa* that was genetically identical to pre-transplant isolates within four weeks post-transplantation, and this colonization could be prevented by topical colistin antibiotic therapy [12]. A different group demonstrated the median time of recovery of *P. aeruginosa* species from CF lung transplant patients was 15 days post-peratively, as compared to 158 days in non-CF recipients. Histologically, evidence of *Pseudomonas* infection was also detected earlier at post-operative day (POD) #10, (vs. POD #261 in non-CF) and at a higher rate (13/44 in CF vs. 3/21 in non-CF) [13]. Overall, although currently available evidence is limited by its retrospective nature and mostly small case series, with many including both surgical and medical controls; however, a correlation between sinonasal and pulmonary health with regards to pathogenic bacterial colonization has been suggested. Thus, ESS plays an important role in reducing the bacterial burden in the upper airway to prevent subsequent seeding of the lower airway.

3. Surgical Management

Although almost all CF patients have endoscopic and radiological findings of sinonasal disease and a majority of them have extensive nasal polyposis, patient-reported subjective symptoms are variable at less than 20% [2]. Despite appropriate medical therapy, 20 to 60% of CF patients go on to require ESS [2]. In a retrospective review, Brook et al. showed that prior history of ESS and severe CFTR mutations are predictive of ESS while Sinonasal Outcome Test (SNOT)-22 score was not [14]. In a different study, CF patients with nasal polyposis, prior history of ESS, lower forced expiratory volume in one second (FEV1), higher Lund-Mackay score, and higher SNOT-22 score was more likely to elect up-front ESS versus medical therapy. Furthermore, a delay in surgery did not affect post-operative improvement [15]. There are no current guidelines specifically for the management of CF CRS, and patient selection for ESS should follow previously established recommendations for the management of CRS [16] with the additional consideration for reducing pulmonary pathogen colonization, especially in post-lung transplant CF patients.

Radiographically, CF patients have a high prevalence of frontal aplasia, and maxillary, ethmoid, and sphenoid hypoplasia. Sclerotic sphenoethmoidal partitions are also commonly found. Interestingly, other important anatomic variants were seen differentially in CF patients: Haller cells and concha bullosa were rarely seen, whereas Onodi cells were more frequently observed [4,17]. Careful pre-operative evaluation of CT findings is critical in avoiding complications and ensuring complete removal of all bony partitions. Complete ESS is especially important in CF CRS, as inspissated secretions may be trapped in partially removed partitions. A recent study also demonstrated high-risk CF mutations are associated with more severe radiographic findings as measured by modified Lund–Mackay scores, as well as higher prevalence of sinus hypoplasia/aplasia [18]. An understanding of CF pathophysiology is important in the surgical management of CF CRS patients to ensure surgical success. In our experience, intra-operative image guidance can be an invaluable tool due to anatomic differences in CF patients, especially in revision cases. However, its use should be judicious and always correlated with knowledge of surgical landmarks. Lastly, a cohort of pediatric CF patients who underwent ESS during and after facial growth spurts was followed prospectively for over 10 years, and no significant differences in cephalometric measurements were demonstrated, which corroborates previous findings on the safety of ESS on pediatric facial growth [19].

Large systematic reviews have demonstrated a definitive benefit of ESS on patient-reported quality of life (QoL) outcomes, while the effect of sinus surgery on pulmonary function tests (PFTs) have yielded conflicting results to date. Khalid et al. demonstrated significant improvement in QoL as measured by the Rhinosinusitis Disability Index (RSDI) in CF patients after ESS that was comparable to control patients, even though CF patients had worse pre-operative CT and endoscopic findings [20]. In one systematic review, Macdonald et al. found that ESS consistently improved sinonasal symptoms in CF patients, and some evidence existed for reduced days of hospitalization for pulmonary exacerbations and usage of intravenous antibiotic therapy. However, no significant changes in pulmonary function tests, including FEV1, were identified [21,22]. Another systematic review similarly demonstrated that ESS led to improved sinonasal symptoms and endoscopic scores, while PFTs were improved in 3/8 level four studies [5]. Kovell et al. demonstrated an improvement in PFTs in pediatric CF patients following ESS, although some of the benefits were mitigated by lower socioeconomic status [23]. Khalfoun and colleagues found that the decline in FEV1 was prevented by ESS in patients with moderate to severe lung disease [8]. Large systematic reviews evaluated the entire aggregate of CF patients; subgroup analysis of high versus low-risk mutations may provide additional insights and can be an area of future research. A study by Halderman and colleagues alluded to this and demonstrated differential responses of PFTs to ESS in homozygous versus heterozygous F5018del CF patients [24].

Endoscopic sinus surgery also plays a critical role in reducing or eradicating pulmonary colonization of pathogens in CF patients. Aanaes and colleagues prospectively followed a cohort of 106 CF patients after ESS with adjuvant systemic and topical therapy, and they demonstrated reduced pulmonary colonization with CF pathogens at 6 months [7]. Furthermore, the percentage of patients without any gram-negative bacteria colonization in the lungs increased from 15% to 33% at 3 years. Although overall pulmonary decline was observed for the cohort, a small percentage of patients had stable lung functions [25]. Holzmann et al. studied the effects of ESS on 37 post-lung transplant CF patients and found a significant correlation between sinus culture positivity and BAL positivity. Successful ESS (defined as less than 3 post-operative sinus aspirates with significant bacterial growth) was associated with significantly reduced incidence of lower airway exacerbations and a trend toward decreased bronchiolitis obliterans syndrome (BOS) [26]. Similarly, Vital et al. demonstrated a significant correlation between chronic sinonasal colonization and lung allograft infection rates in CF patients after lung transplantation and sinus surgery. Furthermore, ESS and daily saline irrigation were successful in eliminating *P. aeruginosa* colonization in more than a third of patients [27]. The absence of persistent airway pathogenic colonization was associated with less frequent and delayed development of BOS and increased overall survival [28]. In contrast, Leung and colleagues found that pre-transplant ESS did not prevent post-transplant *Pseudomonas* re-colonization and did not affect overall survival [29].

4. Extended Sinus Surgery

Recently, modified endoscopic medial maxillectomy (MEMM) has been increasingly performed for recalcitrant maxillary sinus disease. This technique is especially useful in CF patients, allowing large cavities for gravity-dependent drainage, improved topical medication delivery, and access for office-based debridement or polypectomy. A recent study combining MEMM with mucosal stripping of maxillary sinuses and total ethmoidectomy showed significant volume reduction of maxillary sinuses through osteoneogenesis, which the authors proposed as a mechanism for decreased mucus accumulation, thus, chronic bacterial colonization of the sinonasal cavity [30]. The sustained improvement of sinonasal symptoms after MEMM has been demonstrated for up to 6.9 years, although the patient population in this study was more heterogeneous and included all patients with recalcitrant chronic maxillary sinusitis [31].

According to Shatz, a combined Caldwell–Luc approach and medial maxillectomy for CF CRS patients with prior ESS failure were efficacious in reducing episodes of hospitalizations and need for IV antibiotics. Interestingly, FEV1 was significantly improved at 6 months in his cohort of 15 patients [32]. Virgin and colleagues followed a cohort of 22 patients after MEMM and found significant improvement in patient-reported symptom scores, as well as a decreased number of pulmonary exacerbations requiring hospitalization with 1 year follow up [1].

CF patients often have aplastic or hypoplastic frontal sinuses; however, the modified endoscopic Lothrop procedure is a consideration in recalcitrant frontal sinus disease in CF patients. Jaberoo et al. described a series of two CF patients who safely underwent modified Lothrop procedure with good symptomatic improvement [33]. Although the safety and efficacy can be extrapolated from non-CF CRS literature, larger prospective studies are needed to evaluate outcomes of Draf 3 procedures in CF CRS patients.

5. Post-Operative Adjuvant Therapy

Similar to our understanding of non-CF CRS, a combined approach of endoscopic sinus surgery followed by post-surgical adjuvant medical therapy represents the most optimal treatment for disease control in CF CRS. Aanaes et al. demonstrated that intensive post-operative nasal saline irrigation, topical colistin, and office debridement following ESS eradicated pathogenic bacteria in 67% of operated sinuses 6-months post-operatively, with effect sustained up to 3 years [34]. Similarly, the frequency of BAL negativity for CF pathogens increased by 150% 1 year after sinus surgery with adjuvant therapy [7]. Moss and colleagues studied the effect of topical tobramycin irrigation after ESS and found a reduction in the need for future surgical interventions [35]. Combining complete ESS with MEMM and a post-operative regimen that included both oral and topical antibiotic and steroid therapy, Virgin et al. showed a significant reduction of symptoms and hospitalizations for pulmonary exacerbations [1]. Cimmino and colleagues performed a small randomized double-blind placebo-controlled trial of 24 CF patients who underwent sinus surgery and then maintained on dornase alfa therapy, and they demonstrated a significantly improved FEV1 compared to control patients. In addition, patient-reported symptom scores and Lund–Kennedy endoscopic scores were both improved over placebo [36].

6. Summary

The treatment of chronic rhinosinusitis with comorbid cystic fibrosis is complex and challenging. High disease burden found on endoscopic or radiographic examination often does not correlate with patient self-reported symptoms. Currently available data are limited to mostly case series, and further larger prospective studies are much-needed. Endoscopic sinus surgery has been shown to improve sinonasal and pulmonary bacterial colonization, as well as alleviating patient symptoms. The effects of sinus surgery on pulmonary functions are less clear. Despite a paucity of high-quality data and lack of an established treatment algorithm, increasing research has suggested that a multi-disciplinary approach with extensive sinus surgery creating gravity dependent drainage pathways, combined with adjunct topical and medical therapies, offer the most optimal treatment strategy for CF CRS patients.

Funding: This research received no external funding.

Conflicts of Interest: The authors declare no conflict of interest.

References

1. Virgin, F.W.; Rowe, S.M.; Wade, M.B.; Gaggar, A.; Leon, K.J.; Young, K.R.; Woodworth, B.A. Extensive surgical and comprehensive postoperative medical management for cystic fibrosis chronic rhinosinusitis. *Am. J. Rhinol. Allergy* **2012**, *26*, 70–75. [CrossRef] [PubMed]
2. Tipirneni, K.E.; Woodworth, B.A. Medical and Surgical Advancements in the Management of Cystic Fibrosis Chronic Rhinosinusitis. *Curr. Otorhinolaryngol. Rep.* **2017**, *5*, 24–34. [CrossRef]
3. Yang, C.; Chilvers, M.; Montgomery, M.; Nolan, S.J. Dornase alfa for cystic fibrosis. *Cochrane Database Syst. Rev.* **2016**.
4. Orlandi, R.R.; Wiggins, R.H. Radiological Sinonasal Findings in Adults with Cystic Fibrosis. *Am. J. Rhinol.* **2009**, *23*, 307–311. [CrossRef]
5. Liang, J.; Higgins, T.S.; Ishman, S.; Boss, E.F.; Benke, J.R.; Lin, S.Y. Surgical management of chronic rhinosinusitis in cystic fibrosis: A systematic review. *Int. Rhinol.* **2013**, *3*, 814–822. [CrossRef]
6. Illing, E.A.; Woodworth, B.A. Management of the Upper Airway in Cystic Fibrosis. *Curr. Opin. Pulm. Med.* **2014**, *20*, 623–631. [CrossRef]
7. Aanaes, K.; Johansen, H.; Skov, M.; Buchvald, F.; Hjuler, T.; Pressler, T.; Hoiby, N.; Nielsen, K.; Von Buchwald, C. Clinical effects of sinus surgery and adjuvant therapy in cystic fibrosis patients—Can chronic lung infections be postponed? *Rhinol. J.* **2013**, *51*, 222–230. [CrossRef]
8. Khalfoun, S.; Tumin, D.; Ghossein, M.; Lind, M.; Hayes, D., Jr.; Kirkby, S. Improved lung function after sinus susgery in cystic fibrosis patients with moderate obstruction. *Otolaryngol. Head Neck Surg.* **2018**, *158*, 381–385. [CrossRef] [PubMed]
9. Pletcher, S.D.; Goldberg, A.N.; Cope, E.K. Loss of Microbial Niche Specificity between the Upper and Lower Airways in Patients with Cystic Fibrosis. *Laryngoscope* **2018**, *129*, 544–550. [CrossRef]
10. Walter, S.; Gudowius, P.; Bosshammer, J.; Romling, U.; Weissbrodt, H.; Schürmann, W.; Von Der Hardt, H.; Tummler, B. Epidemiology of chronic Pseudomonas aeruginosa infections in the airways of lung transplant recipients with cystic fibrosis. *Thorax* **1997**, *52*, 318–321. [CrossRef] [PubMed]
11. Mainz, J.G.; Naehrlich, L.; Schien, M.; Käding, M.; Schiller, I.; Mayr, S.; Schneider, G.; Wiedemann, B.; Wiehlmann, L.; Cramer, N.; et al. Concordant genotype of upper and lower airways P aeruginosa and S aureus isolates in cystic fibrosis. *Thorax* **2009**, *64*, 535–540. [CrossRef]
12. Mainz, J.G.; Hentschel, J.; Schien, C.; Cramer, N.; Pfister, W.; Beck, J.; Tummler, B. Sinonasal persistence of Pseudomonas aeruginosa after lung transplantation. *J. Cyst. Fibros.* **2012**, *11*, 158–161. [CrossRef]
13. Nunley, D.R.; Grgurich, W.; Iacono, A.T.; Yousem, S.; Ohori, N.P.; Keenan, R.J.; Dauber, J.H. Allograft Colonization and Infections with Pseudomonas in Cystic Fibrosis Lung Transplant Recipients. *Chest* **1998**, *113*, 1235–1243. [CrossRef] [PubMed]
14. Brook, C.D.; Maxfield, A.Z.; Ahmed, H.; Sedaghat, A.R.; Holbrook, E.H.; Gray, S.T. Factors influencing the need for endoscopic sinus surgery in adult patients with cystic fibrosis. *Am. J. Rhinol. Allergy* **2017**, *31*, 44–47. [CrossRef]
15. Ayoub, N.; Thamboo, A.; Habib, A.-R.; Nayak, J.V.; Hwang, P.H.; Habib, A. Determinants and outcomes of upfront surgery versus medical therapy for chronic rhinosinusitis in cystic fibrosis. *Int. Rhinol.* **2017**, *7*, 450–458. [CrossRef]
16. Rosenfeld, R.M.; Piccirillo, J.F.; Chandrasekhar, S.S.; Brook, I.; Ashok Kumar, K.; Kramper, M.; Orlandi, R.R.; Palmer, J.N.; Patel, Z.M.; Peters, A.; et al. Clinical practice guidelines (update): Adult sinusitis. *Otolaryngol. Head Neck Surg.* **2015**, *152*, S1–S39. [CrossRef] [PubMed]
17. Eggesbø, H.; Søvik, S.; Dølvik, S.; Eiklid, K.; Kolmannskog, F. CT characterization of developmental variations of the paranasal sinuses in cystic fibrosis. *Acta Radiol.* **2001**, *42*, 482–493. [CrossRef]

18. Halderman, A.A.; Lee, S.; London, N.R.; Day, A.; Jain, R.; Moore, J.A.; Lin, S.Y. Impact of high- versus low-risk genotype on sinonasal radiographic disease in cystic fibrosis. *Laryngoscope* **2018**, *129*, 788–793. [CrossRef] [PubMed]
19. Van Peteghem, A.; Clement, P. Influence of extensive functional endoscopic sinus surgery (FESS) on facial growth in children with cystic fibrosis. *Int. J. Pediatr. Otorhinolaryngol.* **2006**, *70*, 1407–1413. [CrossRef] [PubMed]
20. Khalid, A.N.; Smith, T.; Mace, J.C. Outcomes of sinus surgery in adults with cystic fibrosis. *Otolaryngol. Neck Surg.* **2009**, *141*, P115. [CrossRef]
21. I MacDonald, K.; Gipsman, A.; Magit, A.; Fandino, M.; Massoud, E.; Witterick, I.J.; Hong, P. Endoscopic sinus surgery in patients with cystic fibrosis: A systematic review and meta-analysis of pulmonary function. *Rhinol. J.* **2012**, *50*, 360–369. [CrossRef]
22. Henriquez, O.A.; Wolfenden, L.L.; Stecenko, A.; DelGaudio, J.M.; Wise, S.K. Endoscopic Sinus Surgery in Adults With Cystic Fibrosis. *Arch. Otolaryngol. Head Neck Surg.* **2012**, *138*, 1167–1170. [CrossRef] [PubMed]
23. Kovell, L.C.; Wang, J.; Ishman, S.L.; Zeitlin, P.L.; Boss, E.F. Cystic fibrosis and sinusitis in children: Outcomes and socioeconomic status. *Otolaryngol. Head Neck Surg.* **2011**, *145*, 146–153. [CrossRef]
24. Halderman, A.A.; West, N.; Benke, J.; Roxbury, C.R.; Lin, S.Y. F508del genotype in endoscopic sinus surgery: Do differences in outcomes exist between genotypic subgroups? *Int. Forum Allergy Rhinol.* **2017**, *7*, 459–466. [CrossRef]
25. Alanin, M.C.; Aanaes, K.; Høiby, N.; Pressler, T.; Skov, M.; Nielsen, K.G.; Taylor-Robinson, D.; Waldmann, E.; Krogh Johansen, H.; von Buchwald, C. Sinus surgery postpones chronic Gram-negative lung infection. *Rhinology* **2016**, *54*, 206–213. [CrossRef] [PubMed]
26. Holzmann, D.; Speich, R.; Kaufmann, T.; Laube, I.; Russi, E.W.; Simmen, D.; Weder, W.; Boehler, A. Effects of sinus surgery in patients with cystic fibrosis after lung transplantation: A 10-year experience. *Transplantation* **2004**, *77*, 134–136. [CrossRef] [PubMed]
27. Vital, D.; Hofer, M.; Boehler, A.; Holzmann, D. Posttransplant sinus surgery in lung transplant recipients with cystic fibrosis: A single institutional experience. *Eur. Arch. Otorhinolaryngol.* **2013**, *270*, 135–159. [CrossRef]
28. Vital, D.; Hofer, M.; Benden, C.; Holzmann, D.; Boehler, A. Impact of Sinus Surgery on Pseudomonal Airway Colonization, Bronchiolitis Obliterans Syndrome and Survival in Cystic Fibrosis Lung Transplant Recipients. *Respiration* **2013**, *86*, 25–31. [CrossRef]
29. Leung, M.-K.; Rachakonda, L.; Weill, D.; Hwang, P.H. Effects of Sinus Surgery on lung Transplantation Outcomes in Cystic Fibrosis. *Am. J. Rhinol.* **2008**, *22*, 192–196. [CrossRef]
30. Buras, M.; Simoncini, A.; Gungor, A. Auto-obliteration of maxillary sinuses through osteogenesis in children with cystic fibrosis: A possible new way to reduce morbidities. *Am. J. Otolaryngol.* **2018**, *39*, 737–740. [CrossRef]
31. Costa, M.L.; Psaltis, A.J.; Nayak, J.V.; Hwang, P.H. Long-term outcomes of endoscopic maxillary mega-antrostomy for refractory chronic maxillary sinusitis. *Int. Forum Allergy Rhinol.* **2015**, *5*, 60–65. [CrossRef] [PubMed]
32. Shatz, A. Management of recurrent sinus disease in children with cystic fibrosis: A combined approach. *Otolaryngol. Head Neck Surg.* **2006**, *135*, 248–252. [CrossRef]
33. Jaberoo, M.C.; Pulido, M.A.; Saleh, H.A. Modified Lothrop procedure in cystic fibrosis patients: Does it have a role? *J. Laryngol. Otol.* **2012**, *127*, 666–669. [CrossRef]
34. Aanaes, K.; Hjuler, T.; Alanin, M.; Von Buchwald, C.; Skov, M.; Johansen, H.K. The Effect of Sinus Surgery with Intensive follow-up on Pathogenic Sinus Bacteria in Patients with Cystic Fibrosis. *Am. J. Rhinol.* **2013**, *27*, e1–e4. [CrossRef]
35. Moss, R.B.; King., V.V. Management of sinusitis in cystic fibrosis by endoscopic surgery and serial antimicrobial lavage. *Arch. Otolaryngol. Head Neck Surg.* **1995**, *121*, 566–572. [CrossRef]
36. Cimmino, M.; Nardone, M.; Cavaliere, M.; Plantulli, A.; Sepe, A.; Esposito, V.; Mazzarella, G.; Raia, V. Dornase Alfa as Postoperative Therapy in Cystic Fibrosis Sinonasal Disease. *Arch. Otolaryngol. Head Neck Surg.* **2005**, *131*, 1097–1101. [CrossRef] [PubMed]

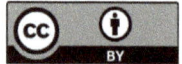

© 2019 by the authors. Licensee MDPI, Basel, Switzerland. This article is an open access article distributed under the terms and conditions of the Creative Commons Attribution (CC BY) license (http://creativecommons.org/licenses/by/4.0/).

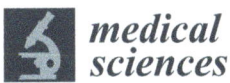

Review

Asthma and Chronic Rhinosinusitis: Diagnosis and Medical Management

Landon Massoth, Cody Anderson and Kibwei A. McKinney *

College of Medicine, University of Oklahoma, Oklahoma City, OK 73104, USA; landon-massoth@ouhsc.edu (L.M.); cody-anderson@ouhsc.edu (C.A.)
* Correspondence: kibwei-mckinney@ouhsc.edu

Received: 21 January 2019; Accepted: 22 March 2019; Published: 27 March 2019

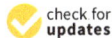

Abstract: Asthma is a prevalent inflammatory condition of the lower airways characterized by variable and recurring symptoms, reversible airflow obstruction, and bronchial hyperresponsiveness (BHR). Symptomatically, these patients may demonstrate wheezing, breathlessness, chest tightness, and coughing. This disease is a substantial burden to a growing population worldwide that currently exceeds 300 million individuals. This is a condition that is frequently encountered, but often overlooked in the field of otolaryngology. In asthma, comorbid conditions are routinely present and contribute to respiratory symptoms, decreased quality of life, and poorer asthma control. It is associated with otolaryngic diseases of the upper airways including allergic rhinitis (AR) and chronic rhinosinusitis (CRS). These conditions have been linked epidemiologically and pathophysiologically. Presently, they are considered in the context of the unified airway theory, which describes the upper and lower airways as a single functional unit. Thus, it is important for otolaryngologists to understand asthma and its complex relationships to comorbid diseases, in order to provide comprehensive care to these patients. In this article, we review key elements necessary for understanding the evaluation and management of asthma and its interrelatedness to CRS.

Keywords: asthma; sinusitis; chronic rhinosinusitis; nasal polyps; eosinophilia; sinus surgery

1. Introduction

Asthma is a prevalent inflammatory condition of the lower airways characterized by variable and recurring symptoms, reversible airflow obstruction, and bronchial hyperresponsiveness (BHR). Symptomatically, these patients may demonstrate wheezing, breathlessness, chest tightness, and coughing. This disease is a substantial burden to a growing population worldwide that currently exceeds 300 million individuals [1]. This is a condition that is frequently encountered, but often overlooked in the field of otolaryngology. In asthma, comorbid conditions are routinely present and contribute to respiratory symptoms, decreased quality of life, and poorer asthma control. It is associated with otolaryngic diseases of the upper airways including allergic rhinitis (AR) and chronic rhinosinusitis (CRS) [2,3]. These conditions have been linked epidemiologically and pathophysiologically. Presently, they are considered in the context of the unified airway theory, which describes the upper and lower airways as a single functional unit [4,5]. Moreover, the upper and lower respiratory tracts share anatomical and histological characteristics. They have common histological structures, including the basement membrane, lamina propria, ciliary epithelium, glands, and goblet cells [6]. Because of these similarities, it is important for otolaryngologists to understand the complex relationships that exist between asthma and comorbid diseases, in order to provide comprehensive care to these patients. In this article, we review key elements necessary for understanding the evaluation and management of asthma and its interrelatedness to CRS.

2. Epidemiology

Asthma is a common condition affecting greater than 4% of the population globally [7]. It is more prevalent in developed countries, and, in particular, the United States [8]. Over the last several decades, there has been a rise in its prevalence. Epidemiologic studies by the Centers for Disease Control (CDC) reported a 3.0% asthma prevalence in the United States in 1970, which rose to 7.8% by 2006 to 2008 [9]. Today, it affects 8.4% of children and 8.1% of adults in the United States [10,11]. It is a leading cause for presentation to the emergency department, accounting for 1.7 million visits in the United States in 2015 [12]. The rate of asthma deaths decreased from 15 per million in 2001 to 10 per million in 2016. Adults were nearly five times more likely than children to die from asthma. There remain gender and racial disparities in morbidity and mortality among different groups. This is demonstrated by the higher death rate among women and non-Hispanic blacks, with the latter group being two to three times more likely to die from asthma when compared with other racial groups [13].

From a pathophysiology standpoint, the current understanding is that certain gene–environment and gene–gene interactions contribute to the development of asthma. Tobacco smoke exposure, pollutants, respiratory viral infections, and obesity are significant risk factors in its pathogenesis [14–17]. Hereditary factors play an apparent role in the development of the disease as well. In a Swedish study, a family history of atopic asthma increased the risk of developing this condition up to four-fold [18]. Moreover, several studies have shown that the offspring of asthmatic parents are at an increased risk of developing asthma [19]. The list of genes associated with asthma continues to grow, as more are elucidated through whole genome sequencing.

Epidemiologic evidence also supports the coexistence of asthma and other upper airway conditions, as previously mentioned. For instance, nearly 80% of patients with asthma report some form of rhinitis, defined as irritation and inflammation of the mucous membranes of the nose. Conversely 10–40% of rhinitis patients report coexistent asthma [20,21]. The presence of rhinitis increases the risk for the development of asthma by three-fold in both atopic and non-atopic individuals [22]. In a study by Linneberg et al., individuals with AR who were sensitized to perennial allergens were found to have a significantly higher likelihood of developing asthma than individuals who were sensitized to seasonal allergens [23].

The prevalence of CRS is estimated to be between 22% and 45% among patients with asthma [24–26]. Among the general population, the prevalence of CRS symptoms is estimated to be 10–12%, with the majority of these patients reporting either moderate or severe symptoms [27]. CRS is associated with more severe asthma, especially in patients with nasal polyps (CRSwNP) [28]. The presence of nasal polyps is similarly associated with more severe sinus symptoms, including facial pain and pressure and hyposmia, relative to CRS without polyps (CRSsNP) [27]. In a recent cluster analysis, performed by the Severe Asthma Research Program (SARP), nearly half of the patients with the most severe burden of disease had a history of previous sinus surgery [26].

3. Pathophysiology of Asthma

The hallmark characteristics of asthma pathogenesis include inflammation of the lower airways through the infiltration of cells, release of potent pro-inflammatory factors, and the remodeling of the airway walls. Allergens, pollutants, irritants, and microbes elicit various inflammatory cascades that are mediated by multiple cell types including dendritic cells, mast cells, eosinophils, T lymphocytes, macrophages, neutrophils, and epithelial cells [29]. These inflammatory influences provoke changes in the respiratory tract, including epithelial shedding, goblet cell hyperplasia, hypertrophy of submucosal mucus glands and bronchial smooth muscle, subepithelial fibrosis with collagen deposition, angiogenesis, and vascular permeability [29]. This is manifested by variable and recurrent episodes of wheezing, breathlessness, chest tightness, and cough. Initially, these changes are reversible with treatment, but with chronic inflammatory insults, irreversible remodeling of the lower airway occurs. These alterations increase the thickness of the airway wall, leading to irreversible airflow obstruction and airway hyperresponsiveness. Similar histopathological changes are often observed in CRS, including mucosal thickening, submucosal gland hypertrophy, collagen deposition, and basement membrane thickening [30].

While inflammation is central to the pathophysiology of asthma, the underlying mechanism is increasingly understood to be multifactorial, reflecting the diversity of the natural history, severity, and treatment responsiveness of the disease. Presently, asthma is seen as an umbrella diagnosis with several distinct mechanistic pathways (endotypes) and variable clinical presentations (phenotypes). While there is little consensus, endotypes in asthma are generally categorized as T-helper type 2 (Th2) cell—high (T2–high) or Th type 2 cell—low (T2–low) [31]. The former is characterized by eosinophilia and atopy, while the latter is manifested by increased neutrophils or a pauci-granulocytic profile. T2–high inflammation is associated with the eosinophilic airway reactivity that is driven by dendritic cell stimulation of Th2 cells and the production of inflammatory cytokines [32]. Allergen exposure leads to the production of Interleukin-33 (IL-33), IL-25, and thymic stromal lymphopoietin (TSLP) by both dendritic and epithelial cells. These mediators, recently classified as alarmins, stimulate Th2 cells to release IL-4, IL-5, and IL-13 that, in turn, stimulate eosinophils, mast cells, and immunoglobulin E (IgE) synthesis through the induction of IgE B cells. Immune memory of IgE responses is then maintained by the development of plasma cells contained in the bone marrow. Recent studies suggest that the respiratory mucosa is the site of development of these cells that maintain immunologic memory of allergen-induced IgE responses [33]. The authors would direct the reader to consider contemporary reviews regarding the biologic development of IgE and immunologic memory in allergic airway disease [33,34].

Nonallergic irritants produce an analogous inflammatory cascade by stimulating the production of IL-33, IL-25, and TSLP, which lead type 2 innate lymphoid cells to produce IL-5 and IL-13. Unlike Th2 cells, type 2 innate lymphoid cells produce little IL-4 and do not elicit an IgE response. Alternatively, in T2–low inflammation, evidence suggests that irritants, pollutants, or infectious agents activate IL-33, IL-23, and IL-6 [35]. IL-33 stimulates the Th17 cell to produce IL-6, IL-17, and IL-8. These cytokines, in turn, trigger neutrophil production. Th17 and Th1 activate neutrophilic inflammation through IL-6, IL-17, interferon gamma, and tumor necrosis factor alpha [35]. A growing understanding of these mechanisms has coincided with the advent of treatment strategies that target specific inflammatory mediators, based on biomarkers that reflect the underlying disease. It is the hope of investigators that further insight will lead to tailored therapy and improved outcomes.

4. Pathophysiology of CRS

The pathogenesis of CRS parallels that of asthma. Specifically, the inflammatory subtypes of CRS mirror T2–high and T2–low inflammatory endotypes observed in asthma [36]. Historically, CRS was categorized as either CRS with nasal polyps or CRS without nasal polyps (CRSsNP), based on the presence or absence of polyps on imaging or sinonasal endoscopy [37]. CRSwNP is generally accepted to have a type 2-predominant inflammatory response, with a predominance of eosinophilic inflammation, including eosinophils, mast cells, elevated IgE, and the expression of type 2 cytokines (IL-4, IL-5, IL-9, IL-13, IL-25, and IL-33). Consequently, CRSwNP has a close association with asthma and other atopic diseases. CRSsNP, on the other hand, is more commonly associated with elevated type 1 cytokines (e.g., interferon-γ), Th-1 helper cells, and a neutrophilic cellular response [37,38]. Recent studies have demonstrated immense heterogeneity between and within these broad phenotypic categories, based on the molecular and cellular pathways that are active in each specific disease state [37–39]. These "endotypes" differ in the severity of disease and demonstrate histopathologic differences in various inflammatory cascades that are the potential targets of therapeutic intervention.

Cluster analyses of the factors contributing to CRS have been performed, taking into consideration the clinical, molecular, and pathological markers of disease [37,40–42]. This has been particularly helpful in differentiating the underlying mechanisms of disease in patients with nasal polyps. Cao et al., for example, found that type 2 immune pathway activation was a predisposing factor toward the development of nasal polyps in both patients with and without eosinophilic inflammation [40].

In another study, Tomassen et al. clustered patients into groups according to their levels of IL-5 expression, as a proxy for the level of eosinophilic inflammation present [43]. In doing so, low levels of IL-5 were shown to have a close association with CRSsNP, while high levels correlated with the highest burden of polyps. Intermediate levels of IL-5 demonstrated variable phenotypic expression of asthma and nasal polyposis, suggesting that there is a subset of CRSwNP patients that exhibits both type 1 and type 2 immune pathway activation [37,38,43]. Nakayama et al. similarly identified disease-specific factors that correlated with clusters of disease, including the presence of perennial allergy, asthma/eosinophilic mucin, and eosinophilic inflammation [44]. In a much larger study of over 100 patients, Soler et al. determined that other patient-related factors were more discriminant in clustering patients with CRSwNP, including age, patient-reported outcome measures (Sinonasal Outcome Test-22 (SNOT-22) scores, productivity loss), and the comorbid presence of fibromyalgia and depression [45]. Ongoing investigation into the relative contributions of patient- and disease-related factors is underway; with the goal of determining how these factors interact to influence the severity of disease and the response to directed therapies.

5. Clinical Features of Asthma

Classically, the cardinal symptoms of asthma include wheezing, breathlessness, chest tightness, and coughing. The clinical features and severity of asthma, however, can vary significantly between individuals and even in a single person over time [46]. Additionally, many asthmatics may only recognize fulminant asthma exacerbation as an indicator of this disease, with a tendency to overlook more subtle, indolent symptoms (e.g., nighttime cough), leading to delays in diagnosis and treatment [47]. Cough associated with asthma classically worsens at night or with activity, is dry, and non-productive. In one Korean study, 680 adult patients were questioned on whether they experience a troublesome cough at night. The association of this symptom with the diagnosis of asthma demonstrated a sensitivity of 62.1%, specificity of 44.8%, positive predictive value (PPV) of 22.8%, and negative predictive value (NPV) of 81.8% [48]. Wheezing is also a common clinical feature of asthma. A large New Zealand study showed that wheezing had a sensitivity of 94% and specificity of 76% for the diagnosis of asthma. Furthermore, this study demonstrated that wheezing with dyspnea was the best predictor of asthma with a sensitivity and specificity of 82% and 90%, respectively [49]. The New Zealand study also examined exercise dyspnea alone. Exercise-induced dyspnea was found to have a sensitivity of 75.4%, specificity of 76.5%, PPV of 22.5%, and NPV of 97.2% [50]. It is, therefore, critical for the otolaryngologist to both inquire about these symptoms and consider further evaluation for asthma when the symptoms present.

Due to the heterogeneity of the disease, a number of asthma phenotypes have been proposed. Phenotypes have been organized according to their association with specific triggers, patient characteristics, or features of clinical presentation. Examples include aspirin sensitivity, adult age of onset, and steroid-resistant subtypes. This heterogeneity prompted the National Heart, Lung, and Blood Institute's Severe Asthma Research Program (SARP) to perform a cluster analysis on adults with mild, moderate, and severe asthma to identify phenotypic clusters which share common traits. The analysis revealed five phenotypic clusters that were predominantly distinguished by lung function and disease age of onset [26]. A similar cluster analysis by SARP identified four phenotypic clusters in children that differed primarily according to asthma duration, the number of asthma controller medications being used, and lung function [51]. Of these clusters, late-onset asthmatics had higher frequency of sinusitis, more severe sinus disease radiographically, and higher rates of sinus surgery [52–54]. Accordingly, it is crucial in these patients to assess for cardinal symptoms associated with CRS, including nasal obstruction, discolored nasal discharge, facial pain or pressure, loss of sense of smell, and cough (in children) that persists for greater than 12 weeks [55,56]. There is growing momentum to pair these clinical phenotypes with pathophysiologic mechanisms. To date, however, the association between clinical phenotype and endotype remains imprecise and, thus, warrants further investigation.

6. Clinical Features of Chronic Rhinosinusitis

Recent studies have demonstrated the immense heterogeneity represented among patients previously categorized under the broad diagnosis CRS with nasal polyps. This has derived from the realization that patients with this phenotype differ in the extent to which tissue and blood eosiniophilia play a role in their pathogenesis. Similar to eosinophilic asthma, eosinophilic chronic rhinosinusitis (eCRS) is associated with aberrant Th2 pathway activation, resulting in activation of the eosinophilic inflammatory cascade and mucociliary dysfunction. These patients tend to manifest a more severe disease presentation, with symptoms that are more refractory to medical and surgical interventions than non-eCRS subtypes. These symptoms include nasal obstruction, olfactory dysfunction, thick mucus drainage, and recurrent episodes of bacterial infection [57].

In a recent review of the literature, Dennis et al. identified four specific classification schema that have been used to endotype patients with CRSwNP. In the type 2 cytokine-based approach, endotypes are differentiated based upon the activation of the Th1 or Th2 pathway. The eosinophil-based approach looks to characterize the endotype of CRSwNP based on the presence of an eosinophilic versus neutrophilic infiltrate within the sinonasal mucosa. This approach accounts for the fact that although these patients manifest a similar phenotype, the degree of eosinophilic inflammation may vary widely between disease processes and among different populations. Eosinophilc mucin, for example, is closely associated with AERD, allergic fungal rhinosinusitis, and eosinophilic mucin chronic rhinosinusitis (EMCRS), but is less often affiliated with non-eosinophilic CRSwNP. A third strategy has looked at the levels of IgE as a marker for different endotypes of CRSwNP. Elevated IgE is noted in all endotypes of patients with polyp disease, with the exception of AERD. However, it is now recognized that local rather than systemic IgE may play a greater role in the development of tissue eosinophilia. More specifically, the production of *Staphylococcus aureus* enterotoxin-specific IgE has been found to correlate more closely with local IgE concentrations and asthma [37,39,43].

Finally, the Cysteinyl Leukotriene (CysLT)-based approach acknowledges aspirin exacerbated respiratory disease (AERD) as a unique clinical phenotype of CRSwNP that is associated with asthma and intolerance of cyclogoxygenase-1 inhibiting agents [37,43,58]. This disease is considered to be a hypersensitivity reaction to acetylsalicylic acid and cyclooxygenase (COX)-1-inhibiting non-steroidal anti-inflammatory drugs that first manifests with nasal congestion and rhinorrhea, typically during the second decade of life. Over several years, it evolves into a more severe and recalcitrant form of disease, that eventually progresses to affect both the upper and lower airways in the form of CRS with nasal polyposis and asthma [59]. The elevated levels of CysLT are due to a functional deficit of COX enzymes and hyperactivity of the 5-lipoxycgenase and leukotriene C4 synthase pathways, resulting in overexpression CystLT [58,59]. A meta-analysis from 2015 found the prevalence of AERD to be 7% in patients with classical asthma and 14% in patients with severe asthma [60]. It also accounts for almost 10% of all patients with CRSwNP [37]. The presence of nasal polyps in a patient with severe asthma should, therefore, prompt the otolaryngologist to consider this particular variant of asthma in their treatment approach.

7. Asthma Diagnosis and Assessment

Asthma can be difficult to diagnose due to its high clinical variability and episodic nature. The diagnosis of asthma is best accomplished through a comprehensive history and physical examination, combined with objective pulmonary function testing [61]. In addition to inquiring about the cardinal symptoms, it is equally important to assess the patient for other risk factors such as smoking, tobacco exposure, family history, and other signs of atopy. Children of parents who are both affected by asthma have an 6.7-fold increased relative risk of asthma when compared to children without any family history [50]. Relying on the physical examination for the diagnosis of asthma also has its challenges. Patients will often present with normal vital signs and physical findings [46]. Moreover, respiratory physical exam findings can be examiner-dependent, as studies have shown only fair-to-good inter-examiner reliability in detecting wheezing on auscultation [62].

Objective pulmonary function testing is considered the gold standard for the definitive diagnosis of asthma. Two findings need to be present with objective diagnostic testing for asthma: (1) the presence of airway obstruction, demonstrated by a decreased forced expiratory volume in one second (FEV1) to forced vital capacity (FVC) ratio, and (2) variability in the severity of airway obstruction when subjected to bronchodilatory or bronchoconstrictive stimuli [61,63]. Spirometry is the objective pulmonary testing method of choice. Using spirometry, an obstructive airway pattern can be established when FEV1/FVC is less than 0.75 in adults or 0.9 in children. Excessive variability in lung function is demonstrated by an increase or decrease of FEV1 greater than 12% after a bronchodilator reversibility test or four week trial of anti-inflammatory treatment [63].

Other supportive testing methods may also be employed. For example, bronchial provocation using exercise or methacholine with measurement of the fractional concentration of exhaled nitric oxide (FeNO) may be employed if the initial spirometry tests are negative and clinical suspicion remains high [46,63]. Additionally, diagnosis of allergic asthma may rely on allergy testing such as skin testing and in vitro ImmunoCAP IgE tests to exclude or confirm the presence of atopy [64]. Finally, a burgeoning area of diagnostic testing is the use of predictive biomarkers in the diagnosis of asthma. Currently, common biomarkers include aberrations in FeNO, serum IgE, sputum and blood eosinophil count, and serum periostin. In particular, FeNO has become more widely available and is a non-invasive reflection of airway eosinophilia. It is useful as a marker of adherence to therapy as well as a predicator of upcoming exacerbation [65]. Recent systematic reviews also demonstrated that tailoring therapy based on FeNO levels may also reduce the number of asthma exacerbations in adults and children [66,67]. Conceptually, the use of biomarkers has the potential advantage of enabling the identification of specific clinical phenotypes and individualizing therapy, with the aim of improving patient outcomes [68].

8. Chronic Rhinosinusitis Diagnosis and Assessment

Chronic sinusitis has been defined as the presence of ≥ 2 of the following symptoms for ≥ 12 weeks duration: anterior or posterior nasal drainage, nasal obstruction, hyposmia or anosmia, and/or facial pain and pressure. These symptoms must be correlated with objective evidence of mucosal disease, including endoscopic evidence of purulence, edema, or nasal polyposis, and/or mucous membrane thickening on computed tomography imaging [55,58].

Although inflammatory markers are helpful, the diagnosis of CRS is still largely contingent upon self-reported symptoms and computed tomography (CT) findings demonstrating polyp disease, mucous membrane thickening, and ostiomeatal obstruction, with the posterior ethmoid and olfactory cleft being the anatomic regions most predictive of this disease process [69]. The Lund–Mackay scoring system has long been used as an objective measure of disease severity, with each sinus being graded on a scale of 0 to 2, based on the degree of mucosal thickening present on CT imaging. The sinuses are grouped into six anatomic regions on each side of the nose, giving a total possible score of 24. These scores provide useful information about the location and extent of diseased tissues, but poorly predict patient symptoms [70]. Self-reported symptoms include the use of validated quality of life surveys, including the SNOT-22 and nasal symptom score (NSS) and rhinosinusitis disability index (RSDI), among many others. While effective as a screening measure, the accuracy of self-reported symptoms is low with a sensitivity and specificity for predicting CRS of 84% and 82%, respectively [71].

Based on the expanding knowledge of CRS endotypes, more research is being done to evaluate the utility of these markers in the diagnosis, work-up, and long-term management of these patients. In addition to the use of IL-5 (which has garnered a great deal of attention due to the proliferation of anti-IL-5 commercially-available monoclonal antibodies), other markers being examined include epithelial-derived cytokines (IL-25 and IL-33), type 2 innate lymphoid cells (ILC2s), cytokines that promote type 2 adaptive responses (IL-4 and IL-13), and the measurement of urinary Leukotriene C4 (LTC$_4$,) in the case of suspected AERD [37–40,43]. Other studies have advocated for the use of structured histopathologic analysis of excised sinonasal tissues, to determine the type of inflammatory infiltrate and the extent of tissue remodeling that may indicate disease severity and predict response to treatment [39]. Among these are basement membrane thickening, subepithelial edema, mucosal ulceration, and fibrosis. To date, none of these histopathologic features have reliably differentiated between the different endotypes of CRS [39].

Similar consideration has been given to utilizing serologic and tissue biomarkers as predictors of disease more globally among all eCRS pathways. Although no strict diagnostic criteria of eCRS exists, it is generally accepted that a tissue eosinophil count >10 per high power field is indicative of this diagnosis. There is growing evidence demonstrating correlations between eCRS severity and inflammatory markers, including blood eosinophilia, eosinophil to total white cell count ratio, and low erythrocyte sedimentation rate [57]. Because of its utility as a marker of lower airway inflammation, FeNO is now being studied as a predictor of eCRS disease severity [72]. Close correlation was found between FeNO and Lund–Mackay CT scores in eCRS patients, whereas FeNO and blood eosinophil count were noted to decrease following functional endoscopic sinus surgery [72]. Of note, there is no increased association between eCRS and serum-specific IgE as measured during immunoCAP testing relative to non-eCRS patients [73]. As mentioned earlier, recent studies have suggested the greater importance of elevated IgE locally, in the pathogenesis of CRS [37,43].

Finally, complimentary testing to identify upper airway disease is essential for asthmatic patients at risk of more severe disease due to the high comorbidity of CRSwNP with asthma [63]. The diagnosis of CRS based on the aforementioned symptom criteria is highly sensitive but inadequately specific [56]. Thus, evaluation must also consist of objective assessment including nasal endoscopy to identify purulence, polyps, or edema or radiographic imaging findings to evaluate for inflammation or mucosal changes within the sinuses [56].

9. Asthma Management

At present, the management of asthma is centered on two concepts: optimizing symptom control and improving objective measures of disease severity. Asthma control consists of the minimization of both daytime and nighttime symptoms, maintenance of a normal level of activity, limiting rescue bronchodilator use, and minimizing untoward events such as severe asthma exacerbations. Severity is the intrinsic intensity of the underlying disease process, which precipitates initial treatment choices and future adjustments. The goal of asthma management is to maintain good symptom control over time with the lowest dose of medications necessary and with the fewest side effects [63]. To achieve this end, a stepwise control-based approach is used, in which pharmacologic treatment is adjusted based on a continuous cycle of assessment, treatment, and review of response [63,74].

Medications for asthma are broadly categorized as long-term control medications, used to achieve and maintain control of persistent asthma, or relieving medications used to treat acute symptoms and exacerbations. Initial controlling medication(s) are selected based on disease severity, which is classified as intermittent, mild persistent, moderate persistent, and severe persistent. For intermittent asthma, short-acting beta-2 agonists (SABA), while not a controlling medication, can be used on an as-needed basis, and can generally control these infrequent symptoms. For mild persistent asthma, low-dose inhaled corticosteroids (ICS) are the cornerstone of treatment. ICS have been shown to reduce asthma symptoms, increase lung function, improve quality of life, and reduce the risk of exacerbations, asthma-related hospitalizations, and death [75–78]. Leukotriene receptor antagonists, while less effective than ICS, can be used in the setting of intolerable adverse effects from ICS, aspirin sensitivity, or with concomitant allergic rhinitis [79–81]. With increasing severity, higher doses of ICS are used along with ICS and long-acting beta-2 agonist (LABA) combination medications. Lastly, patients with persistent symptoms or exacerbations despite optimized therapeutic regimens are considered for add-on treatments that include: long acting muscarinic antagonists (tiotropium), low-dose oral corticosteroids, bronchothermoplasty, and biologic therapy [63]. In particular, the use of several novel biologic agents has resulted in improved lung function, reduced the frequency of severe exacerbations, curtailed use OCS, and improved quality of life in refractory patients with T2-high inflammatory patterns [82–89]. Anti-IgE (Omalizumab) therapy has shown benefit for those with severe allergic asthma [84]. Anti-IL-5 (Mepolizumab, Reslizumab), anti-IL-5 receptor (Benralizumab), and anti-IL-4 receptor (Dupilumab) therapy can be used for treatment of uncontrolled, severe eosinophilic asthma [88,90]. To date, biologic therapies for asthma treatment remain an area of active development. Ongoing investigations seek to determine whether these agents have efficacy in the treatment of patients with CRS with nasal polyps.

As previously noted, the presence of severe asthma should warrant careful consideration of other comorbid conditions [91]. Upper airway comorbid diseases are prevalent in severe asthma, which include: rhinosinusitis, obstructive sleep apnea, vocal cord dysfunction, and gastroesophageal reflux disease. The conditions contribute to worsen asthma control, patient quality of life, and complicate diagnostic assessment and treatment of asthmatic patients [92]. Of particular interest is the treatment of upper airway disease such as allergic rhinitis and chronic rhinosinusitis. Of note, further discussion regarding the impact of management of chronic rhinosinusitis is to follow in a later section. Allergic Rhinitis and its Impact on Asthma (ARIA) evidence-based guidelines recommend the routine use of intranasal corticosteroids (INCS) in patients with allergic asthma [93]. Treatment of rhinitis with INCS has been found to improve asthma outcomes, but only in patients with intermittent disease not receiving ICS [94]. Allergen-specific immunotherapy has been shown to improve symptom severity, reduce the use of medications, and to reduce BHR in mild but not severe asthma [64]. For adult patients with allergic rhinitis and sensitization to house dust mite, persistent asthma requiring ICS (FEV1 > 70%) sublingual allergen immunotherapy (SLIT) can be considered, as it showed benefit in decreasing mild to moderate asthma exacerbations [95].

10. Chronic Rhinosinusitis Management

Given the robust association between asthma and CRS, the question is raised whether treatment of one disease impacts control of the other disease. Medical therapies including saline irrigation, intranasal and systemic glucocorticoids, antibiotics, and anti-leukotriene agents are used in the treatment of CRS with and without nasal polyposis. A placebo-controlled trial of nasal mometasone in patients with CRS and poorly-controlled asthma showed benefit in asthma symptoms with no benefit for asthma outcomes. This suggests that treatment should be targeted to the symptoms of rhinosinusitis, which may contribute to respiratory symptoms, rather than measures that improve asthma control [96].

Biologic agents that have also been studied for the treatment of CRS with NP include omalizumab, mepolizumab, and dupilumab. In a randomized, double-blind, placebo-controlled trial, omalizumab demonstrated improvements in polyp size, Lund–Mackay score, nasal congestion, anterior rhinorrhea, anosmia, wheezing, and dyspnea [38,97]. In another multicenter, double-blind, randomized control trial (RCT) of mepolizumab, Bachert et al. found a reduction in the need for surgery, and improved visual analog scale (VAS) scores of nasal polyposis, endoscopic polyp scores, and self-reported quality of life (SNOT-22) [38,98]. In a similar study design, Bachert also found the use of dupilumab effective in reducing the polyp burden, Lund–Mackay scores, and peak inspiratory flow of CRSwNP patients [99]. Other novel targets currently under investigation include GATA-3, a transcription factor that is active in the production of IL-4, IL-5, and IL-13 in Th2 cells, and the Singlec-8 receptor, which has been shown to induce apoptosis of eosinophils and inhibition of mast cells [37,98,100,101]. Despite this, none of these drugs are yet approved for the treatment of CRS in the United States. In addition, to date, no studies have been performed to examine whether these agents may be used in combination with each other.

With respect to the AERD endotype of CRSwNP, directed therapies have traditionally included the use of leukotriene modifying agents (LTR antagonists and 5-lipoxygenase inhibitors). Aspirin-desensitization therapy and adherence to a low-salicylate diet have also proven to be useful adjunctive measures and are associated with improvement of CysLT and IL-4 levels [102,103]. Despite this, there still remains a subset of patients with AERD in whom these measures are not efficacious, suggesting that there are subendotypes of this disease that warrant further immuno-pathophysiologic characterization [102].

When CRS is recalcitrant to medical therapy, endoscopic sinus surgery (ESS) is considered. Recently, Schlosser et al. demonstrated in a multi-institutional prospective study that patients with pre-existing asthma and CRS experience improved asthma-specific quality of life (QOL) and asthma control after ESS. Chen et al. previously examined asthma control test (ACT) outcomes after ESS and failed to show improvement in mean postoperative ACT scores [104]. Interestingly, the study cohorts differed dramatically in the number of patients that had poorly-controlled asthma, 51% versus 11% respectively. This suggests the benefit of surgery is most evident in patients with poorly-controlled asthma in the pre-operative setting. This is further supported by recent meta-analyses, which found that ESS in patients with concomitant asthma improves clinical asthma outcome measures and objective and subjective nasal outcomes, but fails to show a benefit in pulmonary function testing [105,106]. Recent studies have also reported that early ESS for symptomatic CRS may decrease the development of asthma [107–109]. The otolaryngologist can therefore be of significant help in the difficult-to-treat asthma patient by means of diagnosis and treatment of concordant CRS.

11. Conclusions

Asthma and CRS constitute a group of disorders with varying severity, phenotypic expression, and pathogenesis that are often comorbid and difficult to treat. This review of the literature on their concordance suggests that the optimization of management of each may have a substantial impact on the clinical control of the others. The treatment strategies for concomitant disease are still being elucidated, but novel biologic agents show tremendous promise in preliminary studies. Currently, clinical efforts are best directed at the accurate diagnosis of each condition (including endotyping), symptom control, and disease maintenance through best-practice guidelines for each disease process.

Author Contributions: Conceptualization, L.M. and K.A.M. Writing—original draft preparation, L.M., C.A., and K.A.M. Writing—review and editing, K.A.M.

Funding: This research received no external funding.

Conflicts of Interest: The authors declare no conflicts of interest.

References

1. Masoli, M.; Fabian, D.; Holt, S.; Beasley, R.; Global Initiative for Asthma Program. The Global Burden of Asthma: Executive Summary of the Gina Dissemination Committee Report. *Allergy* **2004**, *59*, 469–478. [CrossRef]
2. Greenberger, P.A. Allergic Rhinitis and Asthma Connection: Treatment Implications. *Allergy Asthma Proc.* **2008**, *29*, 557–564. [CrossRef]
3. Slavin, R.G. The Upper and Lower Airways: The Epidemiological and Pathophysiological Connection. *Allergy Asthma Proc.* **2008**, *29*, 553–556. [CrossRef] [PubMed]
4. Licari, A.; Castagnoli, R.; Denicolo, C.F.; Rossini, L.; Marseglia, A.; Marseglia, G.L. The Nose and the Lung: United Airway Disease? *Front. Pediatr.* **2017**, *5*, 44. [CrossRef] [PubMed]
5. Stachler, R.J. Comorbidities of Asthma and the Unified Airway. *Int. Forum Allergy Rhinol.* **2015**, *5* (Suppl. 1), S17–S22. [CrossRef]
6. Licari, A.; Caimmi, S.; Bosa, L.; Marseglia, A.; Marseglia, G.L.; Caimmi, D. Rhinosinusitis and Asthma: A Very Long Engagement. *Int. J. Immunopathol. Pharmacol.* **2014**, *27*, 499–508. [CrossRef]
7. Bousquet, J.; Dahl, R.; Khaltaev, N. Global Alliance against Chronic Respiratory Diseases. *Allergy* **2007**, *62*, 216–223. [CrossRef]
8. Iqbal, S.; Oraka, E.; Chew, G.L.; Flanders, W.D. Association between Birthplace and Current Asthma: The Role of Environment and Acculturation. *Am. J. Public Health* **2014**, *104* (Suppl. 1), S175–S182. [CrossRef]
9. Loftus, P.A.; Wise, S.K. Epidemiology and Economic Burden of Asthma. *Int. Forum Allergy Rhinol.* **2015**, *5* (Suppl. 1), S7–S10. [CrossRef]

10. Black, L.I.; Benson, V. *Tables of Summary Health Statistics for U.S. Children: 2017*; National Health Interview Survey: Atlanta, GA, USA, 2018.
11. Blackwell, D.L.; Villarroel, M.A. *Tables of Summary Health Statistics for U.S. Adults: 2017*; National Health Interview Survey: Atlanta, GA, USA, 2018.
12. Rui, P.; Kang, K. *National Hospital Ambulatory Medical Care Survey: 2015 Emergency Department Summary Tables*; Centers for Disease Control and Prevention: Atlanta, GA, USA, 2015.
13. Xu, J.; Murphy, S.L.; Kochanek, K.D.; Bastian, B.; Arias, E. Deaths: Final Data for 2016. In *National Vital Statistics Reports*; Centers for Disease Control and Prevention: Atlanta, GA, USA, 2018.
14. Strachan, D.P.; Cook, D.G. Health Effects of Passive Smoking. 6. Parental Smoking and Childhood Asthma: Longitudinal and Case-Control Studies. *Thorax* **1998**, *53*, 204–212. [CrossRef] [PubMed]
15. Jackson, D.J.; Gangnon, R.E.; Evans, M.D.; Roberg, K.A.; Anderson, E.L.; Pappas, T.E.; Printz, M.C.; Lee, W.M.; Shult, P.A.; Reisdorf, E.; et al. Wheezing Rhinovirus Illnesses in Early Life Predict Asthma Development in High-Risk Children. *Am. J. Respir. Crit. Care Med.* **2008**, *178*, 667–672. [CrossRef] [PubMed]
16. Zemp, E.; Elsasser, S.; Schindler, C.; Kunzli, N.; Perruchoud, A.P.; Domenighetti, G.; Medici, T.; Ackermann-Liebrich, U.; Leuenberger, P.; Monn, C.; et al. Long-Term Ambient Air Pollution and Respiratory Symptoms in Adults (Sapaldia Study). The Sapaldia Team. *Am. J. Respir. Crit. Care Med.* **1999**, *159 Pt 1*, 1257–1266. [CrossRef]
17. Beuther, D.A.; Sutherland, E.R. Overweight, Obesity, and Incident Asthma: A Meta-Analysis of Prospective Epidemiologic Studies. *Am. J. Respir. Crit. Care Med.* **2007**, *175*, 661–666. [CrossRef] [PubMed]
18. Lundback, B. Epidemiology of Rhinitis and Asthma. *Clin. Exp. Allergy* **1998**, *28* (Suppl. 2), 3–10.
19. Lim, R.H.; Kobzik, L.; Dahl, M. Risk for Asthma in Offspring of Asthmatic Mothers Versus Fathers: A Meta-Analysis. *PLoS ONE* **2010**, *5*, e10134. [CrossRef] [PubMed]
20. Bousquet, J.; Khaltaev, N.; Cruz, A.A.; Denburg, J.; Fokkens, W.J.; Togias, A.; Zuberbier, T.; Baena-Cagnani, C.E.; Canonica, G.W.; van Weel, C.; et al. Organization World Health, Galen, and AllerGen. Allergic Rhinitis and Its Impact on Asthma (Aria) 2008 Update (in Collaboration with the World Health Organization, Ga(2)Len and Allergen). *Allergy* **2008**, *63* (Suppl. 86), 8–160. [CrossRef]
21. Bousquet, J.; van Cauwenberge, P.; Khaltaev, N. Group Aria Workshop, and Organization World Health. Allergic Rhinitis and Its Impact on Asthma. *J. Allergy Clin. Immunol.* **2001**, *108*, S147–S334. [CrossRef] [PubMed]
22. Guerra, S.; Sherrill, D.L.; Martinez, F.D.; Barbee, R.A. Rhinitis as an Independent Risk Factor for Adult-Onset Asthma. *J. Allergy Clin. Immunol.* **2002**, *109*, 419–425. [CrossRef] [PubMed]
23. Linneberg, A.; Nielsen, N.H.; Frolund, L.; Madsen, F.; Dirksen, A.; Jorgensen, T.; Study Copenhagen Allergy. The Link between Allergic Rhinitis and Allergic Asthma: A Prospective Population-Based Study. The Copenhagen Allergy Study. *Allergy* **2002**, *57*, 1048–1052. [CrossRef] [PubMed]
24. Liou, A.; Grubb, J.R.; Schechtman, K.B.; Hamilos, D.L. Causative and Contributive Factors to Asthma Severity and Patterns of Medication Use in Patients Seeking Specialized Asthma Care. *Chest* **2003**, *124*, 1781–1788. [CrossRef] [PubMed]
25. Ek, A.; Middelveld, R.J.; Bertilsson, H.; Bjerg, A.; Ekerljung, L.; Malinovschi, A.; Stjarne, P.; Larsson, K.; Dahlen, S.E.; Janson, C. Chronic Rhinosinusitis in Asthma Is a Negative Predictor of Quality of Life: Results from the Swedish Ga(2)Len Survey. *Allergy* **2013**, *68*, 1314–1321. [CrossRef]
26. Moore, W.C.; Meyers, D.A.; Wenzel, S.E.; Teague, W.G.; Li, H.; Li, X.; D'Agostino, R., Jr.; Castro, M.; Curran-Everett, D.; Fitzpatrick, A.M.; et al. Identification of Asthma Phenotypes Using Cluster Analysis in the Severe Asthma Research Program. *Am. J. Respir. Crit. Care Med.* **2010**, *181*, 315–323. [CrossRef]
27. Palmer, J.N.; Messina, J.C.; Biletch, R.; Grosel, K.; Mahmoud, R.A. A Cross-Sectional, Population-Based Survey of U.S. Adults with Symptoms of Chronic Rhinosinusitis. *Allergy Asthma Proc.* **2019**, *40*, 48–56. [CrossRef] [PubMed]
28. Hamilos, D.L. Chronic Rhinosinusitis: Epidemiology and Medical Management. *J. Allergy Clin. Immunol.* **2011**, *128*, 693–707. [CrossRef]
29. Fahy, J.V. Type 2 Inflammation in Asthma—Present in Most, Absent in Many. *Nat. Rev. Immunol.* **2015**, *15*, 57–65. [CrossRef] [PubMed]

30. Ponikau, J.U.; Sherris, D.A.; Kephart, G.M.; Kern, E.B.; Gaffey, T.A.; Tarara, J.E.; Kita, H. Features of Airway Remodeling and Eosinophilic Inflammation in Chronic Rhinosinusitis: Is the Histopathology Similar to Asthma? *J. Allergy Clin. Immunol.* **2003**, *112*, 877–882. [CrossRef] [PubMed]
31. Wenzel, S.E.; Schwartz, L.B.; Langmack, E.L.; Halliday, J.L.; Trudeau, J.B.; Gibbs, R.L.; Chu, H.W. Evidence That Severe Asthma Can Be Divided Pathologically into Two Inflammatory Subtypes with Distinct Physiologic and Clinical Characteristics. *Am. J. Respir. Crit. Care Med.* **1999**, *160*, 1001–1008. [CrossRef]
32. Lemanske, R.F., Jr.; Busse, W.W. 6. Asthma. *J. Allergy Clin. Immunol.* **2003**, *111*, S502–S519. [CrossRef] [PubMed]
33. Gould, H.J.; Wu, Y.B. Ige Repertoire and Immunological Memory: Compartmental Regulation and Antibody Function. *Int. Immunol.* **2018**, *30*, 403–412. [CrossRef] [PubMed]
34. Dullaers, M.; de Bruyne, R.; Ramadani, F.; Gould, H.J.; Gevaert, P.; Lambrecht, B.N. The Who, Where, and When of Ige in Allergic Airway Disease. *J. Allergy Clin. Immunol.* **2012**, *129*, 635–645. [CrossRef]
35. Israel, E.; Reddel, H.K. Severe and Difficult-to-Treat Asthma in Adults. *N. Engl. J. Med.* **2017**, *377*, 965–976. [CrossRef] [PubMed]
36. Gurrola, J., 2nd; Borish, L. Chronic Rhinosinusitis: Endotypes, Biomarkers, and Treatment Response. *J. Allergy Clin. Immunol.* **2017**, *140*, 1499–1508. [CrossRef]
37. Dennis, S.K.; Lam, K.; Luong, A. A Review of Classification Schemes for Chronic Rhinosinusitis with Nasal Polyposis Endotypes. *Laryngoscope Investig. Otolaryngol.* **2016**, *1*, 130–134. [CrossRef] [PubMed]
38. Avdeeva, K.; Fokkens, W. Precision Medicine in Chronic Rhinosinusitis with Nasal Polyps. *Curr. Allergy Asthma Rep.* **2018**, *18*, 25. [CrossRef] [PubMed]
39. Shay, A.D.; Tajudeen, B.A. Histopathologic Analysis in the Diagnosis and Management of Chronic Rhinosinusitis. *Curr. Opin. Otolaryngol. Head Neck Surg.* **2019**, *27*, 20–24. [CrossRef]
40. Cao, P.P.; Wang, Z.C.; Schleimer, R.P.; Liu, Z. Pathophysiologic Mechanisms of Chronic Rhinosinusitis and Their Roles in Emerging Disease Endotypes. *Ann. Allergy Asthma Immunol.* **2019**, *122*, 33–40. [CrossRef]
41. Divekar, R.; Rank, M.; Squillace, D.; Kita, H.; Lal, D. Unsupervised Network Mapping of Commercially Available Immunoassay Yields Three Distinct Chronic Rhinosinusitis Endotypes. *Int. Forum Allergy Rhinol.* **2017**, *7*, 373–379. [CrossRef] [PubMed]
42. Shi, L.L.; Xiong, P.; Zhang, L.; Cao, P.P.; Liao, B.; Lu, X.; Cui, Y.H.; Liu, Z. Features of Airway Remodeling in Different Types of Chinese Chronic Rhinosinusitis Are Associated with Inflammation Patterns. *Allergy* **2013**, *68*, 101–109. [CrossRef]
43. Tomassen, P.; Vandeplas, G.; van Zele, T.; Cardell, L.O.; Arebro, J.; Olze, H.; Forster-Ruhrmann, U.; Kowalski, M.L.; Olszewska-Ziaber, A.; Holtappels, G.; et al. Inflammatory Endotypes of Chronic Rhinosinusitis Based on Cluster Analysis of Biomarkers. *J. Allergy Clin. Immunol.* **2016**, *137*, 1449–1456.e4. [CrossRef] [PubMed]
44. Nakayama, T.; Asaka, D.; Yoshikawa, M.; Okushi, T.; Matsuwaki, Y.; Moriyama, H.; Otori, N. Identification of Chronic Rhinosinusitis Phenotypes Using Cluster Analysis. *Am. J. Rhinol. Allergy* **2012**, *26*, 172–176. [CrossRef] [PubMed]
45. Soler, Z.M.; Hyer, J.M.; Ramakrishnan, V.; Smith, T.L.; Mace, J.; Rudmik, L.; Schlosser, R.J. Identification of Chronic Rhinosinusitis Phenotypes Using Cluster Analysis. *Int. Forum Allergy Rhinol.* **2015**, *5*, 399–407. [CrossRef]
46. Reisacher, W.R. Asthma and the Otolaryngologist. *Int. Forum Allergy Rhinol.* **2014**, *4* (Suppl. 2), S70–S73. [CrossRef]
47. Krouse, J.H. Asthma Management for the Otolaryngologist. *Otolaryngol. Clin. North Am.* **2017**, *50*, 1065–1076. [CrossRef] [PubMed]
48. Lim, S.Y.; Jo, Y.J.; Chun, E.M. The Correlation between the Bronchial Hyperresponsiveness to Methacholine and Asthma Like Symptoms by Gina Questionnaires for the Diagnosis of Asthma. *BMC Pulm. Med.* **2014**, *14*, 161. [CrossRef]
49. Sistek, D.; Wickens, K.; Amstrong, R.; D'Souza, W.; Town, I.; Crane, J. Predictive Value of Respiratory Symptoms and Bronchial Hyperresponsiveness to Diagnose Asthma in New Zealand. *Respir. Med.* **2006**, *100*, 2107–2111. [CrossRef]

50. Tarasidis, G.S.; Wilson, K.F. Diagnosis of Asthma: Clinical Assessment. *Int. Forum Allergy Rhinol.* **2015**, *5* (Suppl. 1), S23–S26. [CrossRef]
51. Fitzpatrick, A.M.; Teague, W.G.; Meyers, D.A.; Peters, S.P.; Li, X.; Li, H.; Wenzel, S.E.; Aujla, S.; Castro, M.; Bacharier, L.B.; et al. Heterogeneity of Severe Asthma in Childhood: Confirmation by Cluster Analysis of Children in the National Institutes of Health/National Heart, Lung, and Blood Institute Severe Asthma Research Program. *J. Allergy Clin. Immunol.* **2011**, *127*, 382–389. [CrossRef] [PubMed]
52. Ten Brinke, A.; Grootendorst, D.C.; Schmidt, J.T.; de Bruine, F.T.; van Buchem, M.A.; Sterk, P.J.; Rabe, K.F.; Bel, E.H. Chronic Sinusitis in Severe Asthma Is Related to Sputum Eosinophilia. *J. Allergy Clin. Immunol.* **2002**, *109*, 621–626. [CrossRef] [PubMed]
53. Wu, W.; Bleecker, E.; Moore, W.; Busse, W.W.; Castro, M.; Chung, K.F.; Calhoun, W.J.; Erzurum, S.; Gaston, B.; Israel, E.; et al. Unsupervised Phenotyping of Severe Asthma Research Program Participants Using Expanded Lung Data. *J. Allergy Clin. Immunol.* **2014**, *133*, 1280–1288. [CrossRef]
54. John Staniorski, C.; Price, C.P.E.; Weibman, A.R.; Welch, K.C.; Conley, D.B.; Shintani-Smith, S.; Stevens, W.W.; Peters, A.T.; Grammer, L.; Lidder, A.K.; et al. Asthma Onset Pattern and Patient Outcomes in a Chronic Rhinosinusitis Population. *Int. Forum Allergy Rhinol.* **2018**, *8*, 495–503. [CrossRef]
55. Fokkens, W.J.; Lund, V.J.; Mullol, J.; Bachert, C.; Alobid, I.; Baroody, F.; Cohen, N.; Cervin, A.; Douglas, R.; Gevaert, P.; et al. European Position Paper on Rhinosinusitis and Nasal Polyps 2012. *Rhinology* **2012**, *50* (Suppl. 23), 1–298.
56. Orlandi, R.R.; Kingdom, T.T.; Hwang, P.H.; Smith, T.L.; Alt, J.A.; Baroody, F.M.; Batra, P.S.; Bernal-Sprekelsen, M.; Bhattacharyya, N.; Chandra, R.K.; et al. International Consensus Statement on Allergy and Rhinology: Rhinosinusitis. *Int. Forum Allergy Rhinol.* **2016**, *6* (Suppl. 1), S22–S209. [CrossRef]
57. Ho, J.; Hamizan, A.W.; Alvarado, R.; Rimmer, J.; Sewell, W.A.; Harvey, R.J. Systemic Predictors of Eosinophilic Chronic Rhinosinusitis. *Am. J. Rhinol. Allergy* **2018**, *32*, 252–257. [CrossRef]
58. Orlandi, R.R.; Kingdom, T.T.; Hwang, P.H. International Consensus Statement on Allergy and Rhinology: Rhinosinusitis Executive Summary. *Int. Forum Allergy Rhinol.* **2016**, *6* (Suppl. 1), S3–S21. [CrossRef]
59. Kim, S.D.; Cho, K.S. Samter's Triad: State of the Art. *Clin. Exp. Otorhinolaryngol.* **2018**, *11*, 71–80. [CrossRef]
60. Rajan, J.P.; Wineinger, N.E.; Stevenson, D.D.; White, A.A. Prevalence of Aspirin-Exacerbated Respiratory Disease among Asthmatic Patients: A Meta-Analysis of the Literature. *J. Allergy Clin. Immunol.* **2015**, *135*, 676–681.e1. [CrossRef] [PubMed]
61. Brigham, E.P.; West, N.E. Diagnosis of Asthma: Diagnostic Testing. *Int. Forum Allergy Rhinol.* **2015**, *5* (Suppl. 1), S27–S30. [CrossRef]
62. Benbassat, J.; Baumal, R. Narrative Review: Should Teaching of the Respiratory Physical Examination Be Restricted Only to Signs with Proven Reliability and Validity? *J. Gen. Intern. Med.* **2010**, *25*, 865–872. [CrossRef] [PubMed]
63. Global Initiative for Asthma. *Global Strategy for Asthma Management and Prevention*; Global Initiative for Asthma: Fontana, WI, USA, 2018.
64. Abramson, M.J.; Puy, R.M.; Weiner, J.M. Injection Allergen Immunotherapy for Asthma. *Cochrane Database Syst. Rev.* **2010**, *8*, Cd001186. [CrossRef] [PubMed]
65. Del Giudice, M.M.; Marseglia, G.L.; Leonardi, S.; Tosca, M.A.; Marseglia, A.; Perrone, L.; Ciprandi, G. Fractional Exhaled Nitric Oxide Measurements in Rhinitis and Asthma in Children. *Int. J. Immunopathol. Pharmacol.* **2011**, *24* (Suppl. 4), 29–32. [CrossRef]
66. Petsky, H.L.; Kew, K.M.; Chang, A.B. Exhaled Nitric Oxide Levels to Guide Treatment for Children with Asthma. *Cochrane Database Syst. Rev.* **2016**, *11*, CD011439. [CrossRef] [PubMed]
67. Petsky, H.L.; Kew, K.M.; Turner, C.; Chang, A.B. Exhaled Nitric Oxide Levels to Guide Treatment for Adults with Asthma. *Cochrane Database Syst. Rev.* **2016**, *9*, CD011440. [CrossRef] [PubMed]
68. Medrek, S.K.; Parulekar, A.D.; Hanania, N.A. Predictive Biomarkers for Asthma Therapy. *Curr. Allergy Asthma Rep.* **2017**, *17*, 69. [CrossRef]
69. Sakuma, Y.; Ishitoya, J.; Komatsu, M.; Shiono, O.; Hirama, M.; Yamashita, Y.; Kaneko, T.; Morita, S.; Tsukuda, M. New Clinical Diagnostic Criteria for Eosinophilic Chronic Rhinosinusitis. *Auris Nasus Larynx* **2011**, *38*, 583–588. [CrossRef] [PubMed]

70. Hopkins, C.; Browne, J.P.; Slack, R.; Lund, V.; Brown, P. The Lund-Mackay Staging System for Chronic Rhinosinusitis: How Is It Used and What Does It Predict? *Otolaryngol. Head Neck Surg.* **2007**, *137*, 555–561. [CrossRef]
71. Workman, A.D.; Parasher, A.K.; Blasetti, M.T.; Palmer, J.N.; Adappa, N.D.; Glicksman, J.T. Accuracy of Self-Reported Diagnosis of Chronic Rhinosinusitis. *Otolaryngol. Head Neck Surg.* **2019**, *160*, 556–558. [CrossRef]
72. Kambara, R.; Minami, T.; Akazawa, H.; Tsuji, F.; Sasaki, T.; Inohara, H.; Horii, A. Lower Airway Inflammation in Eosinophilic Chronic Rhinosinusitis as Determined by Exhaled Nitric Oxide. *Int. Arch. Allergy Immunol.* **2017**, *173*, 225–232. [CrossRef]
73. Shah, S.A.; Ishinaga, H.; Takeuchi, K. Pathogenesis of Eosinophilic Chronic Rhinosinusitis. *J. Inflamm.* **2016**, *13*, 11. [CrossRef]
74. National Asthma Education and Prevention Program. *Expert Panel Report Iii: Guidelines for the Diagnosis and Management of Asthma*; National Heart, Lung, and Blood Institute: Bethesda, MD, USA, 2007.
75. O'Byrne, P.M.; Barnes, P.J.; Rodriguez-Roisin, R.; Runnerstrom, E.; Sandstrom, T.; Svensson, K.; Tattersfield, A. Low Dose Inhaled Budesonide and Formoterol in Mild Persistent Asthma: The Optima Randomized Trial. *Am. J. Respir. Crit. Care Med.* **2001**, *164 Pt 1*, 1392–1397. [CrossRef]
76. Suissa, S.; Ernst, P.; Benayoun, S.; Baltzan, M.; Cai, B. Low-Dose Inhaled Corticosteroids and the Prevention of Death from Asthma. *N. Engl. J. Med.* **2000**, *343*, 332–336. [CrossRef]
77. Pauwels, R.A.; Pedersen, S.; Busse, W.W.; Tan, W.C.; Chen, Y.Z.; Ohlsson, S.V.; Ullman, A.; Lamm, C.J.; O'Byrne, P.M.; Start Investigators Group. Early Intervention with Budesonide in Mild Persistent Asthma: A Randomised, Double-Blind Trial. *Lancet* **2003**, *361*, 1071–1076. [CrossRef]
78. Adams, N.P.; Bestall, J.B.; Malouf, R.; Lasserson, T.J.; Jones, P.W. Inhaled Beclomethasone Versus Placebo for Chronic Asthma. *Cochrane Database Syst. Rev.* **2005**, CD002738. [CrossRef]
79. Chauhan, B.F.; Ducharme, F.M. Anti-Leukotriene Agents Compared to Inhaled Corticosteroids in the Management of Recurrent and/or Chronic Asthma in Adults and Children. *Cochrane Database Syst. Rev.* **2012**, *5*, CD002314. [CrossRef] [PubMed]
80. Philip, G.; Nayak, A.S.; Berger, W.E.; Leynadier, F.; Vrijens, F.; Dass, S.B.; Reiss, T.F. The Effect of Montelukast on Rhinitis Symptoms in Patients with Asthma and Seasonal Allergic Rhinitis. *Curr. Med Res. Opin.* **2004**, *20*, 1549–1558. [CrossRef]
81. Dahlen, S.E.; Malmstrom, K.; Nizankowska, E.; Dahlen, B.; Kuna, P.; Kowalski, M.; Lumry, W.R.; Picado, C.; Stevenson, D.D.; Bousquet, J.; et al. Improvement of Aspirin-Intolerant Asthma by Montelukast, a Leukotriene Antagonist: A Randomized, Double-Blind, Placebo-Controlled Trial. *Am. J. Respir. Crit. Care Med.* **2002**, *165*, 9–14. [CrossRef] [PubMed]
82. Busse, W.; Corren, J.; Lanier, B.Q.; McAlary, M.; Fowler-Taylor, A.; Cioppa, G.D.; van As, A.; Gupta, N. Omalizumab, Anti-Ige Recombinant Humanized Monoclonal Antibody, for the Treatment of Severe Allergic Asthma. *J. Allergy Clin. Immunol.* **2001**, *108*, 184–190. [CrossRef] [PubMed]
83. Soler, M.; Matz, J.; Townley, R.; Buhl, R.; O'Brien, J.; Fox, H.; Thirlwell, J.; Gupta, N.; Della Cioppa, G. The Anti-Ige Antibody Omalizumab Reduces Exacerbations and Steroid Requirement in Allergic Asthmatics. *Eur. Respir. J.* **2001**, *18*, 254–261. [CrossRef]
84. Hanania, N.A.; Alpan, O.; Hamilos, D.L.; Condemi, J.J.; Reyes-Rivera, I.; Zhu, J.; Rosen, K.E.; Eisner, M.D.; Wong, D.A.; Busse, W. Omalizumab in Severe Allergic Asthma Inadequately Controlled with Standard Therapy: A Randomized Trial. *Ann. Intern. Med.* **2011**, *154*, 573–582. [CrossRef]
85. Castro, M.; Zangrilli, J.; Wechsler, M.E.; Bateman, E.D.; Brusselle, G.G.; Bardin, P.; Murphy, K.; Maspero, J.F.; O'Brien, C.; Korn, S. Reslizumab for Inadequately Controlled Asthma with Elevated Blood Eosinophil Counts: Results from Two Multicentre, Parallel, Double-Blind, Randomised, Placebo-Controlled, Phase 3 Trials. *Lancet Respir. Med.* **2015**, *3*, 355–366. [CrossRef]
86. Bjermer, L.; Lemiere, C.; Maspero, J.; Weiss, S.; Zangrilli, J.; Germinaro, M. Reslizumab for Inadequately Controlled Asthma with Elevated Blood Eosinophil Levels: A Randomized Phase 3 Study. *Chest* **2016**, *150*, 789–798. [CrossRef]
87. Bleecker, E.R.; FitzGerald, J.M.; Chanez, P.; Papi, A.; Weinstein, S.F.; Barker, P.; Sproule, S.; Gilmartin, G.; Aurivillius, M.; Werkstrom, V.; et al. Efficacy and Safety of Benralizumab for Patients with Severe Asthma Uncontrolled with High-Dosage Inhaled Corticosteroids and Long-Acting Beta2-Agonists (Sirocco): A Randomised, Multicentre, Placebo-Controlled Phase 3 Trial. *Lancet* **2016**, *388*, 2115–2127. [CrossRef]

88. Wenzel, S.; Ford, L.; Pearlman, D.; Spector, S.; Sher, L.; Skobieranda, F.; Wang, L.; Kirkesseli, S.; Rocklin, R.; Bock, B.; et al. Dupilumab in Persistent Asthma with Elevated Eosinophil Levels. *N. Engl. J. Med.* **2013**, *368*, 2455–2466. [CrossRef]
89. Wenzel, S.; Castro, M.; Corren, J.; Maspero, J.; Wang, L.; Zhang, B.; Pirozzi, G.; Sutherland, E.R.; Evans, R.R.; Joish, V.N.; et al. Dupilumab Efficacy and Safety in Adults with Uncontrolled Persistent Asthma Despite Use of Medium-to-High-Dose Inhaled Corticosteroids Plus a Long-Acting Beta2 Agonist: A Randomised Double-Blind Placebo-Controlled Pivotal Phase 2b Dose-Ranging Trial. *Lancet* **2016**, *388*, 31–44. [CrossRef]
90. Wang, F.P.; Liu, T.; Lan, Z.; Li, S.Y.; Mao, H. Efficacy and Safety of Anti-Interleukin-5 Therapy in Patients with Asthma: A Systematic Review and Meta-Analysis. *PLoS ONE* **2016**, *11*, e0166833. [CrossRef] [PubMed]
91. Boulet, L.P. Influence of Comorbid Conditions on Asthma. *Eur. Respir. J.* **2009**, *33*, 897–906. [CrossRef] [PubMed]
92. Licari, A.; Brambilla, I.; de Filippo, M.; Poddighe, D.; Castagnoli, R.; Marseglia, G.L. The Role of Upper Airway Pathology as a Co-Morbidity in Severe Asthma. *Expert Rev. Respir. Med.* **2017**, *11*, 855–865. [CrossRef]
93. Brozek, J.L.; Bousquet, J.; Agache, I.; Agarwal, A.; Bachert, C.; Bosnic-Anticevich, S.; Brignardello-Petersen, R.; Canonica, G.W.; Casale, T.; Chavannes, N.H.; et al. Allergic Rhinitis and Its Impact on Asthma (Aria) Guidelines-2016 Revision. *J. Allergy Clin. Immunol.* **2017**, *140*, 950–958. [CrossRef] [PubMed]
94. Lohia, S.; Schlosser, R.J.; Soler, Z.M. Impact of Intranasal Corticosteroids on Asthma Outcomes in Allergic Rhinitis: A Meta-Analysis. *Allergy* **2013**, *68*, 569–579. [CrossRef] [PubMed]
95. Virchow, J.C.; Backer, V.; Kuna, P.; Prieto, L.; Nolte, H.; Villesen, H.H.; Ljorring, C.; Riis, B.; de Blay, F. Efficacy of a House Dust Mite Sublingual Allergen Immunotherapy Tablet in Adults with Allergic Asthma: A Randomized Clinical Trial. *JAMA* **2016**, *315*, 1715–1725. [CrossRef]
96. American Lung Association-Asthma Clinical Research Centers' Writing Committee; Dixon, A.E.; Castro, M.; Cohen, R.I.; Gerald, L.B.; Holbrook, J.T.; Irvin, C.G.; Mohapatra, S.; Peters, S.P.; Rayapudi, S.; et al. Efficacy of Nasal Mometasone for the Treatment of Chronic Sinonasal Disease in Patients with Inadequately Controlled Asthma. *J. Allergy Clin. Immunol.* **2015**, *135*, 701–709. [CrossRef]
97. Gevaert, P.; Calus, L.; van Zele, T.; Blomme, K.; de Ruyck, N.; Bauters, W.; Hellings, P.; Brusselle, G.; de Bacquer, D.; van Cauwenberge, P.; et al. Omalizumab Is Effective in Allergic and Nonallergic Patients with Nasal Polyps and Asthma. *J. Allergy Clin. Immunol.* **2013**, *131*, 110–116. [CrossRef] [PubMed]
98. Bachert, C.; Sousa, A.R.; Lund, V.J.; Scadding, G.K.; Gevaert, P.; Nasser, S.; Durham, S.R.; Cornet, M.E.; Kariyawasam, H.H.; Gilbert, J. Reduced Need for Surgery in Severe Nasal Polyposis with Mepolizumab: Randomized Trial. *J. Allergy Clin. Immunol.* **2017**, *140*, 1024–1031. [CrossRef] [PubMed]
99. Bachert, C.; Mannent, L.; Naclerio, R.M.; Mullol, J.; Ferguson, B.J.; Gevaert, P.; Hellings, P.; Jiao, L.; Wang, L.; Evans, R.R.; et al. Effect of Subcutaneous Dupilumab on Nasal Polyp Burden in Patients with Chronic Sinusitis and Nasal Polyposis: A Randomized Clinical Trial. *JAMA* **2016**, *315*, 469–479. [CrossRef]
100. Bachert, C.; Zhang, N.; Hellings, P.W.; Bousquet, J. Endotype-Driven Care Pathways in Patients with Chronic Rhinosinusitis. *J. Allergy Clin. Immunol.* **2018**, *141*, 1543–1551. [CrossRef] [PubMed]
101. Schleimer, R.P.; Schnaar, R.L.; Bochner, B.S. Regulation of Airway Inflammation by Siglec-8 and Siglec-9 Sialoglycan Ligand Expression. *Curr. Opin. Allergy Clin. Immunol.* **2016**, *16*, 24–30. [CrossRef] [PubMed]
102. Kowalski, M.L. Heterogeneity of Nsaid-Exacerbated Respiratory Disease: Has the Time Come for Subphenotyping? *Curr. Opin. Pulm. Med.* **2019**, *25*, 64–70. [CrossRef] [PubMed]
103. Sommer, D.D.; Rotenberg, B.W.; Sowerby, L.J.; Lee, J.M.; Janjua, A.; Witterick, I.J.; Monteiro, E.; Gupta, M.K.; Au, M.; Nayan, S. A Novel Treatment Adjunct for Aspirin Exacerbated Respiratory Disease: The Low-Salicylate Diet: A Multicenter Randomized Control Crossover Trial. *Int. Forum Allergy Rhinol.* **2016**, *6*, 385–391. [CrossRef]
104. Chen, F.H.; Zuo, K.J.; Guo, Y.B.; Li, Z.P.; Xu, G.; Xu, R.; Shi, J.B. Long-Term Results of Endoscopic Sinus Surgery-Oriented Treatment for Chronic Rhinosinusitis with Asthma. *Laryngoscope* **2014**, *124*, 24–28. [CrossRef]
105. Vashishta, R.; Soler, Z.M.; Nguyen, S.A.; Schlosser, R.J. A Systematic Review and Meta-Analysis of Asthma Outcomes Following Endoscopic Sinus Surgery for Chronic Rhinosinusitis. *Int. Forum Allergy Rhinol.* **2013**, *3*, 788–794. [CrossRef]
106. Rix, I.; Hakansson, K.; Larsen, C.G.; Frendo, M.; von Buchwald, C. Management of Chronic Rhinosinusitis with Nasal Polyps and Coexisting Asthma: A Systematic Review. *Am. J. Rhinol. Allergy* **2015**, *29*, 193–201. [CrossRef]

107. Benninger, M.S.; Sindwani, R.; Holy, C.E.; Hopkins, C. Impact of Medically Recalcitrant Chronic Rhinosinusitis on Incidence of Asthma. *Int. Forum Allergy Rhinol.* **2016**, *6*, 124–129. [CrossRef] [PubMed]
108. Hopkins, C.; Andrews, P.; Holy, C.E. Does Time to Endoscopic Sinus Surgery Impact Outcomes in Chronic Rhinosinusitis? Retrospective Analysis Using the Uk Clinical Practice Research Data. *Rhinology* **2015**, *53*, 18–24. [CrossRef] [PubMed]
109. Hopkins, C.; Rimmer, J.; Lund, V.J. Does Time to Endoscopic Sinus Surgery Impact Outcomes in Chronic Rhinosinusitis? Prospective Findings from the National Comparative Audit of Surgery for Nasal Polyposis and Chronic Rhinosinusitis. *Rhinology* **2015**, *53*, 10–17. [CrossRef] [PubMed]

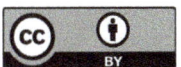

© 2019 by the authors. Licensee MDPI, Basel, Switzerland. This article is an open access article distributed under the terms and conditions of the Creative Commons Attribution (CC BY) license (http://creativecommons.org/licenses/by/4.0/).

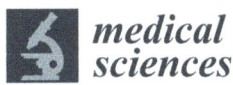

Review

Aspirin Exacerbated Respiratory Disease: Epidemiology, Pathophysiology, and Management

Kevin L. Li, Andrew Y. Lee and Waleed M. Abuzeid *

Department of Otorhinolaryngology: Head and Neck Surgery, Montefiore Medical Center, Albert Einstein College of Medicine, Bronx, NY 10467, USA; keli3@mail.einstein.yu.edu (K.L.L.); andlee@montefiore.org (A.Y.L.)
* Correspondence: wmabuzeid@gmail.com

Received: 19 January 2019; Accepted: 11 March 2019; Published: 17 March 2019

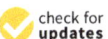

Abstract: The correlation between aspirin sensitivity, asthma, and nasal polyposis was recognized in the early 20th century. Today, this classic triad of symptoms, eponymously named Samter's Triad, is known as aspirin exacerbated respiratory disease (AERD). Aspirin exacerbated respiratory disease affects approximately 0.3–0.9% of the general population in the USA and approximately 7% of asthmatic patients. The management of AERD is challenging as no single modality has proven to have high rates of symptom control. Consequently, disease management typically involves a multimodality approach across both medical and surgical disciplines. This review describes the epidemiology of AERD and the current state-of-the-art as it relates to the underlying pathophysiologic mechanisms of this disease process. A significant proportion of the review is focused on the appropriate diagnostic workup for AERD patients including the utility of aspirin provocation testing. The spectrum of medical treatments, including aspirin desensitization and recently introduced immunotherapies, are discussed in detail. Furthermore, surgical approaches to disease control, including advanced endoscopic techniques, are reviewed and treatment outcomes presented.

Keywords: aspirin exacerbated respiratory disease; AERD; Samter's Triad; chronic rhinosinusitis; endoscopic sinus surgery; aspirin desensitization; nasal polyposis

1. Introduction

Hypersensitivity reactions to aspirin were described as early as 1902 but it was not until 1922 that Widal et al. first described the correlation between aspirin sensitivity, asthma, and nasal polyposis [1]. Subsequently, in 1968, Samter and Beer described the full clinical characteristics of aspirin sensitivity and elucidated the classic triad of symptoms, eponymously named Samter's Triad [1,2]. Samter's Triad is defined as chronic rhinosinusitis with nasal polyposis (CRSwNP), bronchial asthma, and reactions to aspirin or cyclooxygenase-1 (COX-1) inhibitors [3–6]. Since its first description by Widal, there has been considerable literature published on the epidemiology, pathophysiology, and treatment of what is now termed aspirin exacerbated respiratory disease (AERD).

2. Epidemiology

A defining characteristic of AERD is an upper and lower respiratory tract reaction triggered by the ingestion of aspirin (acetylsalicylicacid, ASA) or other COX-1 inhibitors including many non-steroidal anti-inflammatory drugs (NSAIDs) [3,6]. The aspirin or NSAID-induced hypersensitivity reaction results in the rapid onset of symptoms including rhinorrhea, sneezing, nasal congestion, ocular tearing, bronchospasm, skin flushing, hives, and hypotension [7]. It is less common for concurrent respiratory and cutaneous symptoms to occur in patients [8].

It has been difficult to ascertain the prevalence of AERD in the general population [9]. Current estimates suggest that AERD affects approximately 0.3–0.9% of the general population in the USA, with a higher prevalence noted among asthmatic patients (3–20%). A 2014 meta-analysis of clinical trial data demonstrated that AERD was evident in approximately 7% of asthmatic patients [10]. The prevalence of AERD is likely higher in asthmatics who also harbor nasal polyposis with estimates ranging from 30 to 40% [11]. Interestingly, there appears to be a female predominance with incidence ratios of up to 3:2 between females and males, respectively [12]. Furthermore, females tend to have earlier symptom presentation and greater disease severity [5,6]. Generally, AERD manifests in the third or fourth decade of life [13] with much lower rates diagnosed in children [14]. There is no convincing evidence of familial inheritance in AERD [13].

3. Pathophysiology

Aspirin exacerbated respiratory disease is characterized by a non-immunoglobulin E hypersensitivity reaction to ASA/COX-1 inhibitors that is commonly comorbid with but not due to underlying allergic disease [15]. Aspirin exacerbated respiratory disease is thought to be due to abnormalities in arachidonic acid biosynthesis [3,4]. Arachidonic acid can be metabolized through two different pathways: the 5-lipoxygenase (5-LO) pathway and the COX-1 pathway (Figure 1). The 5-LO pathway produces cysteinyl-leukotrienes (Cys-LTs) from arachidonic acid, specifically leukotriene C4, D4, and E4 (LTC4, LTD4, and LTE4) while the COX-1 pathway produces prostacyclins, prostaglandins, and thromboxanes. The underlying defect in AERD is thought to relate to constitutive overproduction of Cys-LTs with a concomitant decrease in downstream products of the COX-1 pathway, the latter of which have an inherent inhibitory effect on Cys-LTs [4,16,17]. The release of this physiologic brake, coupled with Cys-LT overproduction, creates a proinflammatory milieu. Indeed, Cys-LTs have been implicated in the development of rhinitis and AERD through three mechanisms (Figure 2): (1) increased vasodilation and permeability of the nasal vasculature leading to mucosal edema, manifesting clinically as nasal congestion, (2) increased inflammation at the level of the sinonasal epithelium resulting in more mucus production and rhinorrhea, and (3) augmented inflammation through the recruitment of inflammatory cells [16]. The elevated level of Cys-LTs found in the urine, sputum, exhaled breath and peripheral blood of AERD patients supports this theory [3,16]. However, there is still ongoing investigation into the mechanism underlying the constitutive overproduction of Cys-LTs.

To this end, Steinke et al. have further elucidated the roles of interferon-gamma (IFN-γ) and interleukin (IL)-4 in the pathogenesis of AERD. The cytokine milieu in AERD is notable for elevated levels of IFN-γ as compared to asthmatic or eosinophilic sinusitis. This is evidenced by the increased levels of IFN-γ mRNA transcripts and protein. Interferon-gamma is typically associated with a lymphocyte T helper 1 (Th1) response, and the authors postulate that these Th1 cells act to prevent the IgE class-switch recombination, possibly explaining the lack of allergy and atopy in AERD patients [18]. The increased IFN-γ has also been shown to stimulate differentiation of eosinophils through interferon consensus sequence binding protein, a transcription factor, leading to a dramatic upregulation in the number of infiltrating eosinophils [19]. These IFN-γ differentiated eosinophils also have significantly increased levels of LTC4 synthase (LTC4S), possibly explaining the increased levels of Cys-LTs in AERD. Moreover, eosinophils also secrete numerous cytokines and chemokines including IL-4. Both IL-4 and IFN-γ have also been shown to upregulate the Cys-LT1 receptor on multiple cell lines including eosinophils and mast cells (Figure 2) [18,20]. Therefore, IL-4 and IFN-γ both have a role in the constitutive overproduction of Cys-LTs and the overexpression of the Cys-LT1 receptor observed in AERD.

There is growing evidence that AERD may also involve an innate Th2 mucosal immune response and that this response is distinct from allergen-specific etiologies evidenced by AERD occurrence in non-atopic patients who paradoxically show elevated levels of total serum IgE [5,21]. Though there is an eosinophilic predominance in AERD, mast cells may be playing a central role in the observed hypersensitivity reactions. The role of mast cells was first suspected during oral aspirin challenges where a subset of AERD patients showed substantial reductions in FEV1 despite prophylaxis with a Cys-LT1 receptor antagonist while simultaneously showing increased levels of tryptase, a marker of mast cell activation. It has been found that the level of tryptase is inversely correlated with the change in FEV1, and activated mast cells release a host of inflammatory mediators such as prostaglandin D2 (PGD2), which induces inflammation of the respiratory epithelium through recruitment of eosinophils and Th2 cells and also harbors highly bronchoconstrictive properties. Moreover, since these patients were given Cys-LT1 receptor antagonists, the results point towards a potential function for Cys-LTs at other receptors [22–24].

There is increasing evidence for the role of alarmin cytokines such as IL-25, thymic stromal lymphopoeitin (TSLP), and IL-33 in the pathogenesis of the Th2 immune response through activation of group 2 innate lymphoid cells (ILC2s) [25]. Eastman et al. previously demonstrated that ILC2s are both recruited to the nasal mucosa by COX-1 inhibitor induced reactions in AERD patients and are directly correlated with symptom severity [26]. Bucheit et al. found that TSLP also activates mast cells and generates PGD2 in vivo, and in combination with IL-33, led to a synergistic increase in PGD2 production [27]. Interleukin-33 is known to induce activation of mast cells and is typically released from necrotic cells, but infections due to viruses, fungi, and helminthes have also been shown to release IL-33 from epithelial cells [28–30]. Moreover, surgically removed nasal polyps in AERD patients were found to have substantially more IL-33 expression than baseline. Cys-LTs were also found to induce IL-33 expression in murine models, and Pan et al. found that IL-33 stimulates mast cells to generate PGD2, thromboxane B2 (TXB2), and Cys-LTs, and requires COX-1 activity. This suggests that IL-33 could be a bridge between the Cys-LT overexpression and mast cell activation that is typical in AERD and may be a target for future pharmacotherapies [31]. Liu et al. also found that LTE4 is responsible for activation of mast cells through an IL-33 dependent pathway. Previously, LTE4 has been found to cause accumulation of eosinophils, basophils, and Th2 lymphocytes and can directly stimulate Th2 lymphocyte cytokine production [32,33]. Leukotriene E4 stimulation of mast cells has also been shown to substantially upregulate production of PGD2 through both a Cys-LT receptor pathway and a peroxisome proliferator-activated receptor-gamma (PPAR-γ) dependent pathway leading to upregulation of COX-2 (Figure 2) [34].

Laidlaw et al. found that platelet-adherent leukocytes are also effectors of AERD and lead to increased Cys-LT levels. They noted that platelet-adherent eosinophils, neutrophils, and monocytes were markedly increased in AERD patients relative to aspirin-tolerant controls and that urinary LTE4 correlates strongly with the frequency of platelet-adherent neutrophils, eosinophils, and monocytes. Moreover, their experiments found that adherent platelets expressed more than half of the peripheral blood granulocyte LTC4S activity [35]. Previous studies have also shown that activated platelets release arachidonic acid in large quantities and augment 5-LO function through the release of granulocyte macrophage-colony-stimulating factor (GM-CSF) [36,37]. Therefore, the authors concluded that platelets are likely contributing to the basal Cys-LT levels and increased levels of LTC4S found in AERD.

Finally, lipoxins also play an important role in the pathogenesis of AERD [35]. Lipoxins are endogenous anti-inflammatory mediators that typically act to inhibit inflammomodulatory cells and downregulate expression of proinflammatory cytokines such as IFN-γ, IL-5, IL-6, etc. by competing competitively at the Cys-LT1 receptor. Two important lipoxins, LXA4 and LXB4, are generated as a product of arachidonic acid metabolism. It is interesting to note that although there are upregulated Cys-LT1 receptors in patients with AERD, there is a simultaneous downregulation in the production of lipoxins, leading to inadequate competition for receptors with the Cys-LTs [38,39]. Therefore, in AERD, there may be an underlying dysregulation causing deficiency of lipoxins, contributing to the Cys-LT-driven pathophysiology [40].

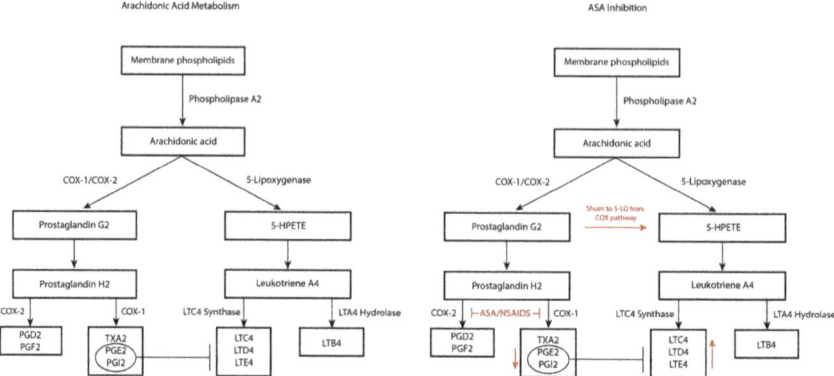

Figure 1. Arachidonic acid pathway (**left panel**) with associated impact of aspirin/non-steroidal anti-inflammatory disease (NSAID) therapy and inhibition (**right panel**). COX-1/2—cyclooxygenase 1/2; PGD2—prostaglandin D2; PGE2—prostaglandin E2; PGF2—prostaglandin F2; PGG2—prostaglandin G2; PGH2—prostaglandin H2; PGI2—prostaglandin I2; TXA2—thromboxane A2; 5-HPETE—5-hydroxyeicosatetranoic acid; LTA4—leukotriene A4; LTB4—leukotriene B4; LTC4—leukotriene C4; LTD4—leukotriene D4; LTE4—leukotriene E4; ASA—acetylsalicylic acid.

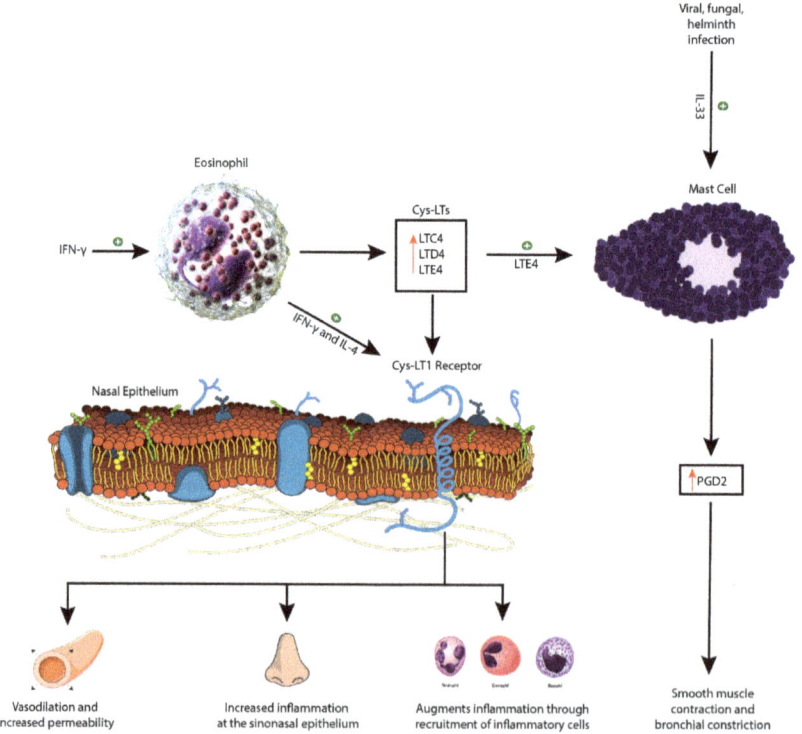

Figure 2. Schematic diagram depicting the role of Cys-LT1 activation and mast cell activation in pathogenesis of aspirin exacerbated respiratory disease (AERD) symptoms. INF-γ—interferon-gamma; IL-4—interleukin-4; Cys-LT—cysteinyl-leukotriene; Cys-LT1—cysteinyl-leukotriene 1; LTC4—leukotriene C4; LTD4—leukotriene D4; LTE4—leukotriene E4; IL-33—interleukin-33; PGD2—prostaglandin D2. This figure incorporates free publicly available images [41–44].

The ingestion of ASA or COX-1 inhibiting NSAIDs by AERD patients further skews Cys-LT production through the inhibition of the COX-1 pathway leading to further shunting of products down the 5-LO pathway [4] (Figure 1). This is evidenced by detection of 5-LO pathway enzyme upregulation in the lungs, sinuses, and nasal polyps in AERD patients, thought to be mostly due to the infiltrating eosinophils and resident mast cells [17]. Furthermore, PGE2 normally has inhibitory effects on eosinophils and mast cells, preventing Cys-LTs from being released. ASA inhibition of PGE2 production additionally skews arachidonic acid production towards the 5-LO pathway.

AERD symptoms tend to develop gradually, beginning with the upper and lower respiratory tract. Typically, nasal congestion and rhinorrhea are the first symptoms. These symptoms persist and progress to hyposmia, nasal polyp formation, and chronic rhinosinusitis (CRS) [12]. On average, asthma developed in patients two years after the initial respiratory tract symptoms appeared, and ASA sensitivity developed within five years of onset [5].

4. Diagnostic Workup

The diagnosis of AERD is made through clinical suspicion and appropriate testing. AERD is suspected if patients have historical upper or lower airway clinical symptoms after ingestion of ASA or NSAIDs, chronic nasal obstruction and watery rhinorrhea, or severe asthma attacks requiring hospitalization with no apparent trigger [45]. Additionally, clinical signs such as nasal polyposis or radiologic findings such as pansinusitis on computed tomography (CT) raise the suspicion for AERD [6]. However, definitive diagnosis is only achieved through ASA provocation testing. The goal of provocation testing is to generate a hypersensitivity reaction in a safe, controlled environment with increasing doses of ASA. These hypersensitivity reactions consist of a constellation of possible symptoms including nasal and ocular itching, sneezing, conjunctivitis, wheezing, coughing, chest tightness, and a drop in forced expiratory volume (FEV1). Additional non-classical symptoms such as laryngeal tightening, stridor, vomiting, urticaria, and angioedema are also possible [13].

There are four types of ASA provocation tests: oral, bronchial, nasal, and intravenous [46]. Oral provocation testing is most commonly used in the US and has a higher sensitivity as compared to the bronchial test. The typical dose of ASA for oral provocation is from 30 to 150 mg (average 60–75 mg) [6]. The bronchial provocation test uses an inhaled L-lysine-ASA and is safer with fewer systemic reactions and is faster to perform compared to the oral challenge. Nasal provocation, typically used in Europe, also uses L-lysine-ASA and is usually reserved for patients who mainly have nasal symptoms or severe asthma contraindicating use of oral or bronchial provocation [46]. Intravenous provocation testing is rarely used outside of Japan. As oral provocation is the most commonly used, its testing protocol will be discussed below.

Provocation testing is classically carried out though accelerated regimens performed over the course of a single day are increasingly being used. In the classic two- or three-day Scripps protocol, a baseline forced expiratory volume in one second (FEV-1) is measured on Day 1 and the challenge is carried out if FEV-1 is at least 70% of the predicted value. Current provocation challenges are commonly preceded by pretreatment with one week of leukotriene modifiers such as montelukast or zileuton. This is due to their efficacy in decreasing the occurrence of severe lower respiratory reactions without inhibiting upper respiratory symptoms. Initial dosing for AERD patients is typically 20 to 40 mg and most bronchial and naso-ocular reactions occur in the dose range of 45 to 100 mg and typically appear within 30–60 min of dosing [47]. A typical oral ASA challenge usually follows a sequential dosing regimen of 30, 45, 60, 100, 150, and 325 mg spaced apart by 3 h. The larger 650 mg dose was found to not elicit additional reactions and has been discontinued from protocols [47].

Forced expiratory volume in one second is measured every 30 min up to 120 min after final dosing and patients are observed for the hypersensitivity reactions mentioned above. A positive reaction is defined as either a decrease in FEV-1 greater than 20% of baseline or if severe extrabronchial hypersensitivity reactions such as profound rhinorrhea and nasal blockade appear, even without a drop in FEV-1 below 20% of baseline. A negative reaction is defined as reaching the maximum dose of ASA without a drop in FEV-1 greater than 20% of baseline or if hypersensitivity symptoms do not appear [46,48]. Provocation tests can also measure urinary LTE4 levels which are correlated with severity of ASA reaction [49]. Increased levels of urinary LTE4 itself is not sufficient for diagnosis of AERD, but when elevated in the context of clinical parameters such as asthma exacerbations and nasal polyposis it nearly doubles the odds of AERD diagnosis [50].

A newer modified challenge protocol utilizes nasal ketorolac before oral ASA challenge and has been shown to be faster than traditional challenge, while still being safe and effective. On Day 1, this challenge protocol gives four escalating doses of ketorolac tromethamine given as nasal sprays 30 min apart with measurement of FEV1 and peak nasal inspiratory flow (PNIF). If symptoms appear, they are treated and the provoking dose is repeated. If no reaction occurs, one hour is allowed to pass before proceeding to oral ASA challenge. The first dose of ASA given is 60 mg and the patient is subsequently monitored for 90 min, wherein if no reaction is elicited, the 60 mg dose is repeated and the patient is monitored for another 90 min. On Day 2, patients are given a 150 mg and a 325 mg dose of ASA spread apart by 3 h. However, if these patients had a reaction to the second 60 mg dose on Day 1, another 60 mg dose is given before proceeding to the 150 mg and 325 mg ASA doses. Most patients finish ASA challenge by the early afternoon on Day 2, considerably faster than traditional ASA challenge testing [51,52]. New ASA challenge protocols are continuing to be developed and increase the efficiency of diagnosis. For example, DeGregorio et al. recently demonstrated that a one-day ASA challenge utilizing a 90-min dose escalation protocol at a starting dose of 40.5 mg was effective in desensitizing AERD patients with stable asthma and baseline FEV-1 greater than or equal to 70% [53].

5. Medical Treatment

The treatment of AERD currently incorporates an algorithm of multiple medical and surgical modalities that progress in a stepwise manner. Treatments include the use of oral and inhaled corticosteroids, leukotriene modifiers, ASA desensitization, and endoscopic sinus surgery [15].

5.1. Corticosteroids

Corticosteroids have been a mainstay therapy for aspirin-tolerant asthma and, although the pathophysiology differs from AERD, both inhaled and systemic corticosteroids have been found to help with subjective and objective symptoms. Specifically, it is useful in treating the symptoms of rhinosinusitis associated with aspirin hypersensitivity. Intranasal corticosteroids like fluticasone propionate have been shown to decrease the number of inflammatory cells including eosinophils and mast cells [54]. A 1997 double-blind crossover, placebo-controlled study focused on the effect of inhaled fluticasone propionate on chronic eosinophilic rhinosinusitis in AERD patients. Outcomes were measured by metrics such as nasal inspiratory peak flow and symptom scores (0–3 points) for morning and evening nasal congestion, rhinorrhea, sneezing and loss of smell. On the last day of the treatment period, L-ASA challenge was repeated. This study found the beneficial effects of fluticasone propionate appeared during the first week and showed a statistically significant increase in nasal inspiratory peak flow and a statistically significant decrease in the nasal symptom scores. The authors also found that fluticasone propionate completely prevented ASA-precipitated nasal reactions in 8 of 13 participants as measured by negative ASA provocation tests in previously positive individuals compared to 2 of 12 in the placebo arm. These results suggest that fluticasone propionate and other topical glucocorticoids are effective in treating rhinosinusitis in AERD [54]. Regardless of route, long-term corticosteroid use is associated with many negative side effects including endocrine, electrolyte, musculoskeletal and neurological disorders [55]. Therefore, other treatment modalities are used in order to reduce the dosage of corticosteroids necessary [56].

5.2. Leukotriene Modifiers

Leukotriene modifiers have also been widely used to treat aspirin-sensitive asthma, and due to the dysregulation of the 5-LO pathway in AERD, these drugs have become an integral treatment option [56]. Typically, anti-leukotrienes such as montelukast work at the level of the Cys-LT1 receptor, acting as a competitive antagonist. This directly leads to decreased production of Cys-LTs, compared to corticosteroids, which do not directly affect the synthesis of leukotrienes [57].

A 2002 multicenter randomized, double-blind, placebo-controlled trial studied the efficacy of montelukast as an additional treatment to AERD in 80 patients, most of whom were already treated with moderate to high doses of corticosteroids. The authors measured FEV-1 and peak expiratory flow rate in addition to asthma symptoms and quality-of-life metrics before and after treatments. The authors noted that improvement from montelukast was observed after one day of treatment. At the end of the trial, FEV-1 showed a statistically significant improvement of 10.2% on average, and patients had an improved peak expiratory flow rate difference of 28 L/min in the morning and 23.1 L/min in the evening. The montelukast arm also showed statistically significant decreases in the number daytime asthma symptoms (12.7%), rescue inhaler use (27.7%), nocturnal awakenings, (35%) and asthma exacerbations (54%). Finally, these patients also experienced significant improvement in the pooled asthma specific quality-of-life questionnaire score. This trial successfully showed that leukotriene antagonists like montelukast improved pulmonary function and asthma control above conventional corticosteroid therapy alone and is a valuable therapy to use in combination with other drug modalities [56].

In addition to montelukast, zileuton and other 5-LO inhibitors have also been studied for therapy in AERD patients. Zileuton directly inhibits 5-LO and offers another method to decrease the production of Cys-LTs. In 1998, a double-blind, placebo-controlled crossover study evaluated the efficacy of zileuton in 40 AERD patients. The patients were well controlled on corticosteroids previously and the zileuton arm received four 600 mg doses. Outcomes measured included FEV-1, peak expiratory flow rate, beta-agonist use, and daytime and nocturnal subjective symptoms, including loss of smell, rhinorrhea, and congestion (scored 0–3). The zileuton arm showed a significant increase in the FEV-1 within hours (12.7% increase, $p < 0.01$) and this benefit lasted throughout the study period. Moreover, there was an 18 L increase in the morning peak expiratory flow rate ($p < 0.001$) compared to placebo, and beta-agonist use decreased by 0.64 puffs ($p < 0.05$). Daytime and nocturnal subjective symptoms scores did not differ significantly in this study, which the authors attribute to the well-controlled symptoms in the patient population at baseline. The authors showed that 5-LO inhibitors were an effective therapy for the treatment of AERD [58]. Interestingly, a clinical questionnaire given to AERD patients found that zileuton is very effective in reducing asthma symptoms compared to montelukast. Moreover, a subgroup analysis in patients with asthma that reported symptoms with ASA use, but were not formally diagnosed, found that zileuton led to a nearly 20% increase in FEV1, indicating that it could be used in the treatment of asthma in AERD patients [59,60]. The efficacy of zileuton over montelukast may be a consequence of its upstream inhibition of 5-lipoxygenase resulting in downregulation of all downstream Cys-LTs, whereas cys-LT1 receptor antagonists, like montelukast, would not significantly affect LTE4 [15,58]. Simultaneous use of a 5-LO inhibitor and a Cys-LT1 receptor antagonist has been suggested but not formally studied at this point [61].

Leukotriene modifiers (both montelukast and zileuton) have also been shown to provide a degree of protection during ASA challenge testing. A 2006 study reviewed the records of 676 patients who completed oral ASA challenges and found that patients taking leukotriene modifiers had significantly less (10–20%) decline in FEV-1 post-provocation. The authors also found that pre-treatment with leukotriene modifiers resulted in less severe asthmatic reactions and a decrease in lower respiratory tract symptoms, possibly due to the abundance of Cys-LT1 receptors in the lower airways compared to the upper airways [61,62]. Consequently, pre-treatment with leukotriene modifiers has been integrated into many ASA challenge protocols.

5.3. Aspirin Desensitization

Corticosteroids and leukotriene modifiers are the first line therapies used to treat AERD. However, if these are insufficient in controlling symptoms, ASA desensitization can provide added benefits.

Some authorities believe that all AERD treatment plans should utilize desensitization [13,63]. The exact mechanism by which ASA desensitization helps control symptoms is currently unknown, but there has been evidence that it decreases IL-4 and STAT6 transcription, decreases production of PGD2, LTE4, and IFN-γ, and decreases the density of Cys-LT receptors [13,17,64–66].

There are multiple protocols developed for ASA desensitization, but typically, ASA desensitization occurs by bringing a patient to a well-equipped clinic and slowly administering increasing doses of ASA until a reaction is elicited [64]. Then, a maintenance dose of 650 mg twice a day is established for continual treatment. If tolerated well, after 6 months, it is reduced to 325 mg twice a day [13,47]. ASA desensitization, followed by either 325 mg twice a day or 650 mg twice a day post-endoscopic sinus surgery with polyp removal is now the standard of care for AERD patients. Typically, the ASA desensitization and treatment is started three to four weeks after the first sinus surgery [15,67].

5.4. Monoclonal Antibodies

Monoclonal antibodies are becoming increasingly popular as a potential therapy in the treatment of AERD. Omalizumab is a recombinant antibody originally designed for treatment of asthma through binding of IgE receptors on mast cells and basophils [68]. Omalizumab has been shown to have mixed efficacy in studies; some authors have found that it displayed rapid clinical effectiveness in reducing mast cell activation and leukotriene overproduction, while others have found that the reduction is not statistically significant [68,69].

In 2013, Gevaert et al. published a randomized, double blind, placebo-controlled trial studying omalizumab in 24 patients with asthma and CRSwNP. The authors had primary end points of polyp size reduction as measured by a total nasal endoscopic polyp score (TPS, scored 0–4). Secondary endpoints were improvement in clinical symptoms measured by Lund-MacKay scores and quality-of-life questionnaire scores including the Short Form Health Questionnaire (SF-36), Rhinosinusitis Outcome Measuring Instrument (RSOM-31), and the Asthma Quality-of-Life Questionnaire (AQLQ). In the omalizumab arm, polyp size and TPS score was significantly reduced by the end of the trial (-2.67, $p = 0.001$), and Lund-Mackay scores were significantly improved as well (17.6 to 13.6, $p = 0.02$) compared to placebo. The omalizumab arm also had significantly improved SF-36 scores for physical health ($p = 0.02$) but not mental health. Rhinosinusitis Outcome Measuring Instrument scores showed significant improvement in sleep ($p = 0.03$) and general symptoms ($p = 0.01$). The mean AQLQ score increased 0.81 ($p = 0.003$). This study demonstrates that omalizumab is capable of improving both disease severity and quality-of-life metrics. Unfortunately, this study primarily focused on CRSwNP and not on AERD. However, within their study group, 12 of 24 patients were given a diagnosis of aspirin hypersensitivity based on medical history. These patients were not challenged with ASA so a definitive diagnosis of AERD could not be given. While further investigation is needed, this could signify a role for omalizumab in AERD patients [70].

In a 2016 prospective cohort study, Hiyashi et al. found that omalizumab administration produced a significant decrease in concentration of urinary LTE4 and a PGD2 metabolite, $9\alpha,11\beta$-prostaglandin F2 (PGD2M) in a post-surgical AERD population and helped to ameliorate upper and lower respiratory tract symptoms, possibly due to mast cell stabilization. Twenty-one patients were studied and, following administration of omalizumab, there was a 76.2% decrease in urinary LTE4 ($p < 0.001$) and an 89% decrease in PGD2M ($p = 0.002$). In addition, they also found a 36.3% drop in eosinophil count ($p = 0.002$) and a significant decrease in the number of exacerbations ($p = 0.002$) and hospitalizations ($p = 0.001$) in a 12-month period. Finally, the Visual Analog Scale (VAS) score was significantly improved for nasal congestion, anterior rhinorrhea, anosmia, dyspnea, wheezing, and cough ($p < 0.001$). The authors demonstrated that omalizumab improved both upper and lower respiratory tract symptoms, which was correlated with the decrease in urinary LTE4 levels [69]. However, this trial was neither randomized nor placebo-controlled, so future studies are needed to verify the potential value of omalizumab in the treatment of AERD.

Mepolizumab is another monoclonal antibody that has been proposed as therapy for AERD. Mepolizumab targets IL-5 and was originally designed to treat eosinophilic asthma, but Gevaert et al. found in a randomized, double-blind placebo-controlled study in CRSwNP patients that injection of two 750 mg doses significantly reduced the total polyp score (-1.30, $p = 0.028$) and showed improved CT scan results in 12 of 20 patients when reviewed by three separate raters (Fleiss κ = 0.679) [71–73]. Again, this study was not specifically designed for AERD patients but 5/20 patients in the treatment group had aspirin sensitivity. Bachert et al. found in a similar randomized, double-blind, placebo-controlled study with 107 CRSwNP patients that 750 mg of mepolizumab every four weeks for six doses resulted in a significant reduction in the endoscopic nasal polyposis score (50% of patients improved by >1 point), and the odds ratio of having a reduction in total endoscopic nasal polyp score was high (6.6, $p = 0.025$). The nasal polyposis severity VAS score was also significantly improved for rhinorrhea ($p < 0.001$), mucus in throat ($p < 0.001$), nasal blockage ($p = 0.002$), and loss of smell ($p < 0.001$). There was also significant improvement in the Sino-Nasal Outcome Test (SNOT-22) scores (42 to 27.1, $p = 0.005$). The authors concluded that administration of mepolizumab decreased the overall need for surgical intervention [74]. This study was also not stratified to include AERD patients and is not directly applicable to this patient population. However, a 2018 retrospective study on mepolizumab for AERD patients has shown some positive results. Fourteen AERD patients at Brigham and Women's Hospital, Boston, MA, USA, who received at least three doses of mepolizumab were included in the study and outcomes such as absolute eosinophil count (AEC), SNOT-22, asthma control test (ACT) scores, and FEV1 were investigated. At baseline, many of these patients had already received numerous AERD treatments such as polypectomies, high-dose aspirin, and oral glucocorticoids. After receiving at least three doses of mepolizumab, the AEC decreased significantly ($p < 0.01$), SNOT-22 decreased by 17.7 points ($p < 0.01$), ACT score increased significantly by 5.1 ($p = 0.002$), but FEV1 percent predicted increased non-significantly by 6.3% ($p = 0.16$). Additionally, no patient required sinus surgery during this time and no patient needed to start or increased their dose of glucocorticoids. On the contrary, five of the seven patients on oral glucocorticoids actually reduced their doses and two of five patients on daily-inhaled corticosteroids/long-acting beta-agonists were able to reduce their doses as well. This was the first study to show the efficacy of mepolizumab in AERD patients, but future double-blinded, controlled studies are needed to confirm this data [75]. Reslizumab and benralizumab are similar agents that also target IL-5 and may have similar efficacy but further investigation is needed to fully elucidate the effectiveness for AERD patients [71].

Dupilumab is the latest monoclonal antibody studied as a therapy for CRSwNP. It is a fully humanized monoclonal antibody that acts directly against the IL-4 receptor α subunit. This in turn inhibits the action of both IL-4 and IL-13, two cytokines that are integral to the Th2-cell mediated inflammatory response. Dupilumab has already been shown to be effective in treating patients with atopic dermatitis and asthma [76]. In a multicenter, randomized, double-blind placebo-controlled parallel-group study conducted in the US and Europe, Wenzel et al. studied dupilumab treatment of CRSwNP refractory to intranasal corticosteroids alone in 104 patients, 15 of which were aspirin sensitive. They found that dupilumab resulted in significant improvements in endoscopic, radiographic, clinical, and pharmacological measures 16 weeks post-treatment. The primary end point was number of asthma exacerbations, and dupilumab showed a significantly reduced number of exacerbations compared to placebo (odds ratio 0.08, $p < 0.001$). Additionally, FEV1 improved by 0.27 L compared to placebo ($p < 0.001$) and morning peak expiratory flow improved by 34.6 L/min compared to placebo ($p = 0.005$). They also found significant improvement in quality-of-life metrics like SNOT-22 (-8.49, $p = 0.003$) with improved sense of smell, fewer symptoms of nasal obstruction and decreased nighttime awakenings. The authors demonstrated that dupilumab treatment in persistent asthma was associated with fewer exacerbations and increased objective and subjective outcome metrics. This improvement was seen in a population that was already treated with medium to high doses of inhaled glucocorticoids and long-acting beta agonists, further suggesting that blocking IL-4 and IL-13 signaling results in an improvement in nasal polyposis, asthma, and improved upper and lower respiratory tract inflammation [77]. A substudy on AERD patients in a phase II trial of dupilumab by Mullol et al. showed that treatment with dupilumab produced an improvement in almost 10 items in the University of Pennsylvania Smell Identification Test (UPSIT) and led to a 30 point reduction in SNOT-22 score, as well as a 2.5 point reduction in Total Polyp Score [78]. Although there is a lack of studies specifically on AERD patients, future studies may prove dupilumab to be a valuable therapeutic agent [76].

6. Surgical Procedures and Outcomes

The role of endoscopic sinus surgery (ESS) can play an integral part in treatment of AERD patients, having a role in decreasing disease burden itself while providing an opportunity for more effective medical treatment [79]. Surgical approaches are targeted towards optimizing the ventilation and drainage of the paranasal sinuses through the widening of the sinus ostia and removal of inflamed bone and soft tissue components. Critically, surgery also enhances the delivery of topical corticosteroids into the paranasal sinuses thereby improving control of inflammation at the level of the sinus epithelium. Computational fluid dynamic models have shown generally enhanced delivery of sinus rinses into the paranasal sinuses after ESS with one study predicting a 10-fold increase in the number of nebulized particles deposited within the maxillary sinus after uncinectomy and antrostomy [80,81]. Furthermore, a separate study evaluating a cohort of 28 patients with confirmed AERD by aspirin challenge, found that that AERD patients were less reactive to an aspirin challenge 3–4 weeks after endoscopic sinus surgery with 43% ($p < 0.001$) having no detectable reaction [82].

AERD patients are known to be a particularly difficult patient population to successfully manage and in whom single modality treatment is rarely successful with quoted failure rates of up to 90% for standard endoscopic sinus surgery [3,83]. Most commonly, dual therapy with a surgical approach combined with ASA desensitization is implemented rather than single modality therapy. The use of sinus surgery leads to decreases in symptomatic severity providing an optimal window in which to proceed with additional treatments including aspirin desensitization and therapy. The ideal time period post-surgical intervention has been postulated as 2–4 weeks [84].

The combined method has shown an improvement in both subjective and objective measures of sinonasal outcomes as measured by SNOT scores [63,85]. In the retrospective review conducted by Cho et al. examining outcomes of aspirin desensitization post-ESS in AERD patients, the authors noted that SNOT-22 scores significantly decreased immediately postoperatively at one week ($p = 0.042$) and four weeks ($p = 0.046$) and continued to remain low through the 30-month post-desensitization follow up period. Endoscopic polyp grade also decreased significantly in the post-operative period ($p < 0.001$) and remained low for up to 30 months post-desensitization with no significant recurrence of polyp burden [85]. This may imply that long-term aspirin desensitization may prevent or slow the progression of the inflammatory process within the sinuses [86]. In a study examining long-term clinical outcomes of ASA desensitization therapy, 92 patients completed a questionnaire regarding nasal symptoms during/after ASA desensitization therapy that was initiated 5–10 years prior with 68% of patients not requiring further sinus surgery and 85% of patients finding it helpful in improving airway disease and quality of life. Interestingly, within this same cohort, ASA therapy did not reduce the total number of sinus surgeries ($p = 0.56$) or delay time to the next sinus/polyp surgery ($p = 0.27$) in those that required further interventions [87]. However, another study found that after surgery, ASA desensitization and long-term ASA therapy reduced reoperative intervention from an average of once every three years to once every 10 years. This further emphasizes the importance of ASA desensitization in combination with surgery [88].

Compared to patients with non-AERD CRSwNP, AERD patients tend to have more severe sinonasal symptoms, as measured on validated symptom score surveys, and a higher incidence of recurrent polyposis up to as high as 90% [83], resulting in higher rates of surgical intervention [45,63,89]. On average, AERD patients undergo 2.6 endoscopic sinus surgeries during their lifetime and tend to be younger at the time of first surgery [90]. When comparing AERD CRSwNP to non-AERD CRSwNP (asthma + CRSwNP and CRSwNP alone), one study—the design of which was predicated on the interpretation of disease severity based on a diagnostic CT scan—demonstrated that 66% of AERD CRSwNP patients were classified as having severe sinus disease compared to 23% and 10% in the other groups, respectively ($p < 0.001$) [90]. In addition to more aggressive symptoms, patients with AERD have significantly worse surgical outcomes compared to patients with non-AERD sinus disease [91]. In a cohort of 549 patients with nasal polyposis undergoing ESS, patients with AERD had increased odds of requiring a second surgery for recurrence compared to patients without asthma or asthma alone (odds ratio 2.7, $p < 0.01$) [83]. There has been no conclusive randomized trial data driving the choice for surgical treatment of AERD, and as such, multiple surgical techniques and procedures have been developed to treat CRS and AERD refractory to medical treatment [63,92]. In the past few decades, the surgical approach has evolved from invasive procedures to minimally invasive endoscopic mucosal-sparing surgeries [93]. Some authors suggest a graduated approach to surgical intervention that is tailored to the patient's disease process and severity. Factors that help with this personalized approach include the patient's disease history, nasal endoscopy, and CT findings [92,94].

6.1. Functional Endoscopic Sinus Surgery

The standard of management for CRS and AERD refractory to medical treatment is functional endoscopic sinus surgery (FESS) [95,96]. The primary goal is to clear diseased tissue within the sinonasal cavities under endoscopic guidance, to re-establish ventilation and drainage via normal physiologic routes, and to optimize the delivery of topical therapeutics, particularly corticosteroids, to the epithelium of the paranasal sinuses [97]. For patients with refractory CRS after initial primary FESS, there are advanced surgical procedures used to treat the frontal, maxillary, or ethmoid sinuses which are discussed below [93].

Functional endoscopic sinus surgery alone in the noncomplicated CRS patient has yielded significant improvements in quality-of-life metrics but, in AERD patients, the role of surgery is less definitive. Surgical intervention alone in the AERD cohort has shown initial improvements in symptoms and disease control but with high rates of recurrence and need for subsequent surgeries [83]. In one study looking at complete ESS, entailing surgical access to all paranasal sinuses, versus targeted ESS, which involves treating only those sinuses that appear diseased on preoperative CT imaging, ASA sensitivity was an independent predictor for complete ESS. Furthermore, complete ESS showed greater improvements in quality-of-life metrics compared to the targeted therapy cohort [98].

The true impact of ESS within the AERD cohort is best characterized when used in conjunction with aspirin desensitization as this is the optimal use scenario based on our current understanding of disease management. In a retrospective review of 32 patients undergoing complete ESS followed by aspirin desensitization therapy, only three patients (9.4%) needed revision sinus surgery within the 30 month follow-up period—one of these patients had stopped ASA therapy during the course of the study [89]. Furthermore, overall SNOT-22 scores showed significant improvement one month postoperatively compared to preoperative baseline (47.0 vs. 15.2, $p < 0.001$) and remained statistically unchanged during the 30 month follow-up period after ASA desensitization was initiated, consistent with previous studies [85,89]. Complete ESS has a role in treatment of AERD patients with significant initial improvement in disease burden and quality-of-life measures, but the evidence thus far suggests that combining complete ESS with ASA desensitization post-operatively produces the greatest effect on disease control.

6.2. Endoscopic Modified Lothrop Procedure/Draf 3

Frontal sinus surgery has high treatment failure rates and often requires revision surgery. One study found that ethmoidectomy without frontal sinusotomy could be used as a first-step procedure for treatment of chronic frontal sinusitis in patients who are already on maximal medical therapy. However, nasal polyposis and ASA sensitivity were independent risk factors predicting failure in those who underwent treatment with this more conservative ethmoidectomy alone approach [99].

This suggests that ethmoidectomy alone may be inadequate for treatment of frontal sinus disease within high-risk recurrent groups such as AERD patients.

An alternative to salvage failed FESS is the endoscopic modified Lothrop procedure (EMLP), also known as the Draf 3 procedure [93,95]. Endoscopic modified Lothrop procedure results in a large common drainage pathway for both frontal sinuses by removing the medial frontal sinus floor bilaterally to the orbits laterally and resecting the superior nasal septum and intersinus septum [94,100]. Another advantage is the ability for sinus rinses to penetrate and distribute within the frontal sinus through the new common pathway with mathematical models showing a significantly increased penetration of sinus rinses into the frontal sinuses after EMLP [101]. Naidoo et al. found in a retrospective cohort study that EMLP allows for increased delivery of topical steroids to control local mucosal inflammation as well as increasing the ventilation into the frontal sinuses. Unfortunately, there appears to be a subset of patients that have exacerbations despite long-term medical therapy [96].

A 2018 meta-analysis by Abuzeid et al. showed that EMLP improved symptoms in 82.3% of patients with 75.9% of patients reporting improvement when EMLP was used as a salvage surgery after failure of primary FESS. Interestingly, the authors found that patients with ASA sensitivity and asthma appeared to have a lower incidence of reoperation, which was attributed to possible evolution to a more aggressive surgical technique based on an understanding that AERD patients were at higher risk of surgical failure [95]. Nevertheless, failure rates in EMLP have been cited as 5–21% across diverse patient pathologies, with many of these cases then requiring a revision EMLP or frontal sinus obliteration [91,96,102]. Failure typically occurred secondary to recurrent polyposis or stenosis of the ostium [91]. Generally, EMLP is considered a safe and efficacious surgery in the modern era. Furthermore, EMLP provides an attractive option for revision surgery as it does not preclude additional surgical options should patients develop refractory disease [95,102].

6.3. Complete Total Ethmoidectomy with Mucosal Stripping

In AERD patients, complete total ethmoidectomy with mucosal stripping or nasalization has been shown to have greater efficacy than conventional ethmoidectomy [93]. Nasalization involves the systematic removal of all the bony lamellae and mucosa in the ethmoid sinuses followed by maxillary antrostomy, sphenoidotomy, frontal sinusotomy, and middle turbinectomy [93].

Eloy et al. found that patients who underwent nasalization showed superior improvement in nasal symptoms compared to those who underwent a standard ESS and the outcomes were more durable. Specifically, olfactory improvement in the nasalization arm lasted for three years compared to only two years of symptom improvement in the ethmoidectomy group [93]. Jankowski et al. has also shown that nasalization is superior with regards to overall symptoms, disease severity as measured on CT, and endoscopic appearance of the post-operative mucosa. Immediately post-operative, patients were started on nasal lavages and local beclomethasone sprays. Critically, nasal polyp recurrence rate was 22.7% in the nasalization arm versus 58.3% in patients undergoing traditional ethmoidectomy. When performed by a skilled sinus surgeon, nasalization was not found to be more hazardous than standard ethmoidectomy [103].

7. Conclusions

Treatment of CRSwNP in the setting of AERD poses a challenging problem within the otolaryngology community. With higher rates of refractory disease despite optimal medical and surgical treatment options, finding the right combination of treatment modalities to help improve symptom control and quality-of-life within this patient population continues to be an active area of research interest. Further improvements in disease control will likely hinge on modification of the underlying inflammatory milieu at the level of the sinonasal epithelium. This will involve the continued development and introduction of biologic immunomodulators for clinical use. Advanced FESS procedures will also play an increasing role in optimizing the delivery of medical therapies and directly modifying the levels of inflammation in the sinuses. Continued advances in these areas, and a better understanding of the ideal timing for specific interventions, will lead to an era of patient-specific treatment and, potentially, improved long-term disease control.

Author Contributions: W.M.A.; Investigation: K.L.L.; Writing—Original Draft Preparation: K.L.L.; Writing—Review and Editing: A.Y.L. and W.M.A.; Supervision: W.M.A.

Funding: This research received no external funding.

Conflicts of Interest: The authors declare no conflicts of interest.

References

1. Widal, F.; Abrami, P.; Lermoyez, J. First complete description of the aspirin idiosyncrasy-asthma-nasal polyposis syndrome (plus urticaria)–1922 (with a note on aspirin desensitization). *J. Asthma* **1987**, *24*, 297–300. [PubMed]
2. Samter, M.; Beers, R.F., Jr. Intolerance to aspirin. Clinical studies and consideration of its pathogenesis. *Ann. Intern. Med.* **1968**, *68*, 975–983. [CrossRef]
3. Sakalar, E.G.; Muluk, N.B.; Kar, M.; Cingi, C. Aspirin-exacerbated respiratory disease and current treatment modalities. *Eur. Arch. Otorhinolaryngol.* **2017**, *274*, 1291–1300. [CrossRef] [PubMed]
4. Kim, S.D.; Cho, K.S. Samter's Triad: State of the Art. *Clin. Exp. Otorhinolaryngol.* **2018**, *11*, 71–80. [CrossRef] [PubMed]
5. Szczeklik, A.; Nizankowska, E.; Duplaga, M. Natural history of aspirin-induced asthma. AIANE Investigators. European Network on Aspirin-Induced Asthma. *Eur. Respir. J.* **2000**, *16*, 432–436. [CrossRef] [PubMed]
6. Szczeklik, A.; Stevenson, D.D. Aspirin-induced asthma: Advances in pathogenesis, diagnosis, and management. *J. Allergy Clin. Immunol.* **2003**, *111*, 913–921. [CrossRef] [PubMed]
7. Gudziol, V.; Michel, M.; Sonnefeld, C.; Koschel, D.; Hummel, T. Olfaction and sinonasal symptoms in patients with CRSwNP and AERD and without AERD: A cross-sectional and longitudinal study. *Eur. Arch. Otorhinolaryngol.* **2017**, *274*, 1487–1493. [CrossRef] [PubMed]
8. Lumry, W.R.; Curd, J.G.; Zeiger, R.S.; Pleskow, W.W.; Stevenson, D.D. Aspirin-sensitive rhinosinusitis: The clinical syndrome and effects of aspirin administration. *J. Allergy Clin. Immunol.* **1983**, *71*, 580–587. [CrossRef]
9. Stevenson, D.; Szczeklik, A. Clinical and pathologic perspectives on aspirin sensitivity and asthma. *J. Allergy Clin. Immunol.* **2006**, *118*, 773–786. [CrossRef] [PubMed]
10. Rajan, J.P.; Wineinger, N.E.; Stevenson, D.D.; White, A.A. Prevalence of aspirin-exacerbated respiratory disease among asthmatic patients: A meta-analysis of the literature. *J. Allergy Clin. Immunol.* **2015**, *135*, 676–681.e1. [CrossRef] [PubMed]
11. Jenkins, C.; Costello, J.; Hodge, L. Systematic review of prevalence of aspirin induced asthma and its implications for clinical practice. *BMJ* **2004**, *328*, 434. [CrossRef] [PubMed]
12. Berges-Gimeno, M.P.; Simon, R.A.; Stevenson, D.D. The natural history and clinical characteristics of aspirin-exacerbated respiratory disease. *Ann. Allergy Asthma Immunol.* **2002**, *89*, 474–478. [CrossRef]
13. White, A.A.; Stevenson, D.D. Aspirin-exacerbated respiratory disease: Update on pathogenesis and desensitization. *Semin. Respir. Crit. Care Med.* **2012**, *33*, 588–594. [CrossRef]
14. Kidon, M.I.; Kang, L.W.; Chin, C.W.; Hoon, L.S.; See, Y.; Goh, A.; Lin, J.T.; Chay, O.M. Early presentation with angioedema and urticaria in cross-reactive hypersensitivity to nonsteroidal antiinflammatory drugs among young, Asian, atopic children. *Pediatrics* **2005**, *116*, e675–e680. [CrossRef] [PubMed]
15. White, A.A.; Stevenson, D.D. Aspirin-Exacerbated Respiratory Disease. *N. Engl. J. Med.* **2018**, *379*, 1060–1070. [CrossRef]
16. Peters-Golden, M.; Gleason, M.M.; Togias, A. Cysteinyl leukotrienes: Multi-functional mediators in allergic rhinitis. *Clin. Exp. Allergy* **2006**, *36*, 689–703. [CrossRef]
17. Steinke, J.W.; Borish, L. Factors driving the aspirin exacerbated respiratory disease phenotype. *Am. J. Rhinol. Allergy* **2015**, *29*, 35–40. [CrossRef]
18. Steinke, J.W.; Liu, L.; Huyett, P.; Negri, J.; Payne, S.C.; Borish, L. Prominent role of IFN-gamma in patients with aspirin-exacerbated respiratory disease. *J. Allergy Clin. Immunol.* **2013**, *132*, 856–865.e3. [CrossRef]
19. Milanovic, M.; Terszowski, G.; Struck, D.; Liesenfeld, O.; Carstanjen, D. IFN consensus sequence binding protein (Icsbp) is critical for eosinophil development. *J. Immunol.* **2008**, *181*, 5045–5053. [CrossRef]

20. Mellor, E.A.; Austen, K.F.; Boyce, J.A. Cysteinyl leukotrienes and uridine diphosphate induce cytokine generation by human mast cells through an interleukin 4-regulated pathway that is inhibited by leukotriene receptor antagonists. *J. Exp. Med.* **2002**, *195*, 583–592. [CrossRef]
21. Johns, C.B.; Laidlaw, T.M. Elevated total serum IgE in nonatopic patients with aspirin-exacerbated respiratory disease. *Am. J. Rhinol. Allergy* **2014**, *28*, 287–289. [CrossRef]
22. Cahill, K.N.; Murphy, K.; Singer, J.; Israel, E.; Boyce, J.A.; Laidlaw, T.M. Plasma tryptase elevation during aspirin-induced reactions in aspirin-exacerbated respiratory disease. *J. Allergy Clin. Immunol.* **2019**, *143*, 799–803.e2. [CrossRef] [PubMed]
23. Cahill, K.N.; Bensko, J.C.; Boyce, J.A.; Laidlaw, T.M. Prostaglandin D(2): A dominant mediator of aspirin-exacerbated respiratory disease. *J. Allergy Clin. Immunol.* **2015**, *135*, 245–252. [CrossRef] [PubMed]
24. Hirai, H.; Tanaka, K.; Yoshie, O.; Ogawa, K.; Kenmotsu, K.; Takamori, Y.; Ichimasa, M.; Sugamura, K.; Nakamura, M.; Takano, S.; et al. Prostaglandin D2 selectively induces chemotaxis in T helper type 2 cells, eosinophils, and basophils via seven-transmembrane receptor CRTH2. *J. Exp. Med.* **2001**, *193*, 255–261. [CrossRef] [PubMed]
25. Cavagnero, K.; Doherty, T.A. Cytokine and Lipid Mediator Regulation of Group 2 Innate Lymphoid Cells (ILC2s) in Human Allergic Airway Disease. *J. Cytokine Biol.* **2017**, *2*. [CrossRef]
26. Eastman, J.J.; Cavagnero, K.J.; Deconde, A.S.; Kim, A.S.; Karta, M.R.; Broide, D.H.; Zuraw, B.L.; White, A.A.; Christiansen, S.C.; Doherty, T.A. Group 2 innate lymphoid cells are recruited to the nasal mucosa in patients with aspirin-exacerbated respiratory disease. *J. Allergy Clin. Immunol.* **2017**, *140*, 101–108.e3. [CrossRef]
27. Buchheit, K.M.; Cahill, K.N.; Katz, H.R.; Murphy, K.C.; Feng, C.; Lee-Sarwar, K.; Lai, J.; Bhattacharyya, N.; Israel, E.; Boyce, J.A.; et al. Thymic stromal lymphopoietin controls prostaglandin D2 generation in patients with aspirin-exacerbated respiratory disease. *J. Allergy Clin. Immunol.* **2016**, *137*, 1566–1576.e5. [CrossRef] [PubMed]
28. Jackson, D.J.; Makrinioti, H.; Rana, B.M.; Shamji, B.W.; Trujillo-Torralbo, M.B.; Footitt, J.; Jerico, D.-R.; Telcian, A.G.; Nikonova, A.; Zhu, J.; et al. IL-33-dependent type 2 inflammation during rhinovirus-induced asthma exacerbations in vivo. *Am. J. Respir. Crit. Care Med.* **2014**, *190*, 1373–1382. [CrossRef] [PubMed]
29. Snelgrove, R.J.; Gregory, L.G.; Peiro, T.; Akthar, S.; Campbell, G.A.; Walker, S.A.; Lloyd, C.M. Alternaria-derived serine protease activity drives IL-33-mediated asthma exacerbations. *J. Allergy Clin. Immunol.* **2014**, *134*, 583–592.e6. [CrossRef]
30. Hung, L.Y.; Lewkowich, I.P.; Dawson, L.A.; Downey, J.; Yang, Y.; Smith, D.E.; Herbert, D.R. IL-33 drives biphasic IL-13 production for noncanonical Type 2 immunity against hookworms. *Proc. Natl. Acad. Sci. USA* **2013**, *110*, 282–287. [CrossRef]
31. Liu, T.; Kanaoka, Y.; Barrett, N.A.; Feng, C.; Garofalo, D.; Lai, J.; Buchheit, K.; Bhattacharya, N.; Laidlaw, T.M.; Katz, H.R.; et al. Aspirin-Exacerbated Respiratory Disease Involves a Cysteinyl Leukotriene-Driven IL-33-Mediated Mast Cell Activation Pathway. *J. Immunol.* **2015**, *195*, 3537–3545. [CrossRef]
32. Austen, K.F.; Maekawa, A.; Kanaoka, Y.; Boyce, J.A. The leukotriene E4 puzzle: Finding the missing pieces and revealing the pathobiologic implications. *J. Allergy Clin. Immunol.* **2009**, *124*, 406–414; quiz 415–416. [CrossRef] [PubMed]
33. Xue, L.; Gyles, S.L.; Wettey, F.R.; Gazi, L.; Townsend, E.; Hunter, M.G.; Pettipher, R. Prostaglandin D2 causes preferential induction of proinflammatory Th2 cytokine production through an action on chemoattractant receptor-like molecule expressed on Th2 cells. *J. Immunol.* **2005**, *175*, 6531–6536. [CrossRef]
34. Paruchuri, S.; Jiang, Y.; Feng, C.; Francis, S.A.; Plutzky, J.; Boyce, J.A. Leukotriene E4 activates peroxisome proliferator-activated receptor gamma and induces prostaglandin D2 generation by human mast cells. *J. Biol. Chem.* **2008**, *283*, 16477–16487. [CrossRef]
35. Laidlaw, T.M.; Kidder, M.S.; Bhattacharyya, N.; Xing, W.; Shen, S.; Milne, G.L.; Castells, M.C.; Chhay, H.; Boyce, J.A. Cysteinyl leukotriene overproduction in aspirin-exacerbated respiratory disease is driven by platelet-adherent leukocytes. *Blood* **2012**, *119*, 3790–3798. [CrossRef] [PubMed]
36. Antoine, C.; Murphy, R.C.; Henson, P.M.; Maclouf, J. Time-dependent utilization of platelet arachidonic acid by the neutrophil in formation of 5-lipoxygenase products in platelet-neutrophil co-incubations. *Biochim. Biophys. Acta* **1992**, *1128*, 139–146. [CrossRef]
37. Raiden, S.; Schettini, J.; Salamone, G.; Trevani, A.; Vermeulen, M.; Gamberale, R.; Giordano, M.; Geffner, J. Human platelets produce granulocyte-macrophage colony-stimulating factor and delay eosinophil apoptosis. *Lab. Investig.* **2003**, *83*, 589–598. [CrossRef] [PubMed]

38. Serhan, C.N.; Chiang, N.; Van Dyke, T.E. Resolving inflammation: Dual anti-inflammatory and pro-resolution lipid mediators. *Nat. Rev. Immunol.* **2008**, *8*, 349–361. [CrossRef] [PubMed]
39. Narayanankutty, A.; Resendiz-Hernandez, J.M.; Falfan-Valencia, R.; Teran, L.M. Biochemical pathogenesis of aspirin exacerbated respiratory disease (AERD). *Clin. Biochem.* **2013**, *46*, 566–578. [CrossRef]
40. Laidlaw, T.M.; Boyce, J.A. Pathogenesis of aspirin-exacerbated respiratory disease and reactions. *Immunol. Allergy Clin. N. Am.* **2013**, *33*, 195–210. [CrossRef]
41. Human Nose. Available online: http://pngimg.com/uploads/nose/nose_PNG2.png (accessed on 12 March 2019).
42. Mast Cell. Hematopoiesis (Human) Diagram en. Available online: https://commons.wikimedia.org/wiki/File:Mast_cell.svg (accessed on 12 March 2019).
43. Art, S.M. Vasodilation. Available online: https://smart.servier.com/smart_image/vasodilation/ (accessed on 12 March 2019).
44. Physiology, A. 1907 Granular Leukocytes. Connexions Web Site. Available online: http://cnx.org/content/col11496/1.6/ (accessed on 12 March 2019).
45. Szczeklik, A.; Nizankowska, E. Clinical features and diagnosis of aspirin induced asthma. *Thorax* **2000**, *55* (Suppl. 2), S42–S44. [CrossRef]
46. Nizankowska-Mogilnicka, E.; Bochenek, G.; Mastalerz, L.; Swierczynska, M.; Picado, C.; Scadding, G.; Kowalski, M.L.; Setkowicz, M.; Ring, J.; Brockow, K.; et al. EAACI/GA2LEN guideline: Aspirin provocation tests for diagnosis of aspirin hypersensitivity. *Allergy* **2007**, *62*, 1111–1118. [CrossRef]
47. Hope, A.P.; Woessner, K.A.; Simon, R.A.; Stevenson, D.D. Rational approach to aspirin dosing during oral challenges and desensitization of patients with aspirin-exacerbated respiratory disease. *J. Allergy Clin. Immunol.* **2009**, *123*, 406–410. [CrossRef] [PubMed]
48. Nizankowska, E.; Bestynska-Krypel, A.; Cmiel, A.; Szczeklik, A. Oral and bronchial provocation tests with aspirin for diagnosis of aspirin-induced asthma. *Eur. Respir. J.* **2000**, *15*, 863–869. [CrossRef]
49. Nasser, S.M.; Patel, M.; Bell, G.S.; Lee, T.H. The effect of aspirin desensitization on urinary leukotriene E4 concentrations in aspirin-sensitive asthma. *Am. J. Respir. Crit. Care Med.* **1995**, *151*, 1326–1330. [CrossRef] [PubMed]
50. Bochenek, G.; Stachura, T.; Szafraniec, K.; Plutecka, H.; Sanak, M.; Nizankowska-Mogilnicka, E.; Sladek, K. Diagnostic Accuracy of Urinary LTE4 Measurement to Predict Aspirin-Exacerbated Respiratory Disease in Patients with Asthma. *J. Allergy Clin. Immunol. Pract.* **2018**, *6*, 528–535. [CrossRef] [PubMed]
51. Lee, R.U.; White, A.A.; Ding, D.; Dursun, A.B.; Woessner, K.M.; Simon, R.A.; Stevenson, D.D. Use of intranasal ketorolac and modified oral aspirin challenge for desensitization of aspirin-exacerbated respiratory disease. *Ann. Allergy Asthma Immunol.* **2010**, *105*, 130–135. [CrossRef]
52. Scott, D.R.; White, A.A. Approach to desensitization in aspirin-exacerbated respiratory disease. *Ann. Allergy Asthma Immunol.* **2014**, *112*, 13–17. [CrossRef]
53. DeGregorio, G.A.; Singer, J.; Cahill, K.N.; Laidlaw, T. A 1-Day, 90-Minute Aspirin Challenge and Desensitization Protocol in Aspirin-Exacerbated Respiratory Disease. *J. Allergy Clin. Immunol. Pract.* **2018**. [CrossRef] [PubMed]
54. Mastalerz, L.; Milewski, M.; Duplaga, M.; Nizankowska, E.; Szczeklik, A. Intranasal fluticasone propionate for chronic eosinophilic rhinitis in patients with aspirin-induced asthma. *Allergy* **1997**, *52*, 895–900. [CrossRef]
55. Sarnes, E.; Crofford, L.; Watson, M.; Dennis, G.; Kan, H.; Bass, D. Incidence and US costs of corticosteroid-associated adverse events: A systematic literature review. *Clin. Ther.* **2011**, *33*, 1413–1432. [CrossRef] [PubMed]
56. Dahlen, S.E.; Malmstrom, K.; Nizankowska, E.; Dahlen, B.; Kuna, P.; Kowalski, M.; Lumry, W.R.; Picado, C.; Stevenson, D.D.; Bousquet, J.; et al. Improvement of aspirin-intolerant asthma by montelukast, a leukotriene antagonist: A randomized, double-blind, placebo-controlled trial. *Am. J. Respir. Crit. Care Med.* **2002**, *165*, 9–14. [CrossRef] [PubMed]
57. De Lepeleire, I.; Reiss, T.F.; Rochette, F.; Botto, A.; Zhang, J.; Kundu, S.; Decramer, M. Montelukast causes prolonged, potent leukotriene D4-receptor antagonism in the airways of patients with asthma. *Clin. Pharmacol. Ther.* **1997**, *61*, 83–92. [CrossRef]

58. Dahlen, B.; Nizankowska, E.; Szczeklik, A.; Zetterstrom, O.; Bochenek, G.; Kumlin, M.; Mastalerz, L.; Pinis, G.; Swanson, L.J.; Boodhoo, T.I.; et al. Benefits from adding the 5-lipoxygenase inhibitor zileuton to conventional therapy in aspirin-intolerant asthmatics. *Am. J. Respir. Crit. Care Med.* **1998**, *157*, 1187–1194. [CrossRef] [PubMed]
59. Ta, V.; White, A.A. Survey-Defined Patient Experiences With Aspirin-Exacerbated Respiratory Disease. *J. Allergy Clin. Immunol. Pract.* **2015**, *3*, 711–718. [CrossRef] [PubMed]
60. Laidlaw, T.M.; Fuentes, D.J.; Wang, Y. Efficacy of Zileuton in Patients with Asthma and History of Aspirin Sensitivity: A Retrospective Analysis of Data from Two Phase 3 Studies. *J. Allergy Clin. Immunol.* **2017**, *139*, AB384. [CrossRef]
61. White, A.; Ludington, E.; Mehra, P.; Stevenson, D.D.; Simon, R.A. Effect of leukotriene modifier drugs on the safety of oral aspirin challenges. *Ann. Allergy Asthma Immunol.* **2006**, *97*, 688–693. [CrossRef]
62. Heise, C.E.; O'Dowd, B.F.; Figueroa, D.J.; Sawyer, N.; Nguyen, T.; Im, D.S.; Stocco, R.; Bellefeuille, J.N.; Abramovitz, M.; Cheng, R.; et al. Characterization of the human cysteinyl leukotriene 2 receptor. *J. Biol. Chem.* **2000**, *275*, 30531–30536. [CrossRef]
63. Adelman, J.; McLean, C.; Shaigany, K.; Krouse, J.H. The Role of Surgery in Management of Samter's Triad: A Systematic Review. *Otolaryngol. Head Neck Surg.* **2016**, *155*, 220–237. [CrossRef]
64. Xu, J.J.; Sowerby, L.; Rotenberg, B.W. Aspirin desensitization for aspirin-exacerbated respiratory disease (Samter's Triad): A systematic review of the literature. *Int. Forum Allergy Rhinol.* **2013**, *3*, 915–920. [CrossRef]
65. Bobolea, I.; Del Pozo, V.; Sanz, V.; Cabanas, R.; Fiandor, A.; Alfonso-Carrillo, C.; Salcedo, M.A.; Heredia Revuelto, R.; Quirce, S. Aspirin desensitization in aspirin-exacerbated respiratory disease: New insights into the molecular mechanisms. *Respir. Med.* **2018**, *143*, 39–41. [CrossRef] [PubMed]
66. Arm, J.P.; O'Hickey, S.P.; Spur, B.W.; Lee, T.H. Airway responsiveness to histamine and leukotriene E4 in subjects with aspirin-induced asthma. *Am. Rev. Respir. Dis.* **1989**, *140*, 148–153. [CrossRef] [PubMed]
67. Stevenson, D.D.; Simon, R.A. Selection of patients for aspirin desensitization treatment. *J. Allergy Clin. Immunol.* **2006**, *118*, 801–804. [CrossRef] [PubMed]
68. Lang, D.M.; Aronica, M.A.; Maierson, E.S.; Wang, X.F.; Vasas, D.C.; Hazen, S.L. Omalizumab can inhibit respiratory reaction during aspirin desensitization. *Ann. Allergy Asthma Immunol.* **2018**, *121*, 98–104. [CrossRef]
69. Hayashi, H.; Mitsui, C.; Nakatani, E.; Fukutomi, Y.; Kajiwara, K.; Watai, K.; Sekiya, K.; Tsuburai, T.; Akiyama, K.; Hasegawa, Y.; et al. Omalizumab reduces cysteinyl leukotriene and 9alpha,11beta-prostaglandin F2 overproduction in aspirin-exacerbated respiratory disease. *J. Allergy Clin. Immunol.* **2016**, *137*, 1585–1587.e4. [CrossRef] [PubMed]
70. Gevaert, P.; Calus, L.; Van Zele, T.; Blomme, K.; De Ruyck, N.; Bauters, W.; Hellings, P.; Brusselle, G.; De Bacquer, D.; van Cauwenberge, P.; et al. Omalizumab is effective in allergic and nonallergic patients with nasal polyps and asthma. *J. Allergy Clin. Immunol.* **2013**, *131*, 110–116.e1. [CrossRef] [PubMed]
71. Henriksen, D.P.; Bodtger, U.; Sidenius, K.; Maltbaek, N.; Pedersen, L.; Madsen, H.; Andersson, E.A.; Norgaard, O.; Madsen, L.K.; Chawes, B.L. Efficacy, adverse events, and inter-drug comparison of mepolizumab and reslizumab anti-IL-5 treatments of severe asthma - a systematic review and meta-analysis. *Eur. Clin. Respir. J.* **2018**, *5*, 1536097. [CrossRef] [PubMed]
72. Gevaert, P.; Van Bruaene, N.; Cattaert, T.; Van Steen, K.; Van Zele, T.; Acke, F.; De Ruyck, N.; Blomme, K.; Sousa, A.R.; Marshall, R.P.; et al. Mepolizumab, a humanized anti-IL-5 mAb, as a treatment option for severe nasal polyposis. *J. Allergy Clin. Immunol.* **2011**, *128*, 989–995.e8. [CrossRef]
73. Chupp, G.L.; Bradford, E.S.; Albers, F.C.; Bratton, D.J.; Wang-Jairaj, J.; Nelsen, L.M.; Trevor, J.L.; Magnan, A.; Ten Brinke, A. Efficacy of mepolizumab add-on therapy on health-related quality of life and markers of asthma control in severe eosinophilic asthma (MUSCA): A randomised, double-blind, placebo-controlled, parallel-group, multicentre, phase 3b trial. *Lancet Respir. Med.* **2017**, *5*, 390–400. [CrossRef]
74. Bachert, C.; Sousa, A.R.; Lund, V.J.; Scadding, G.K.; Gevaert, P.; Nasser, S.; Durham, S.R.; Cornet, M.E.; Kariyawasam, H.H.; Gilbert, J.; et al. Reduced need for surgery in severe nasal polyposis with mepolizumab: Randomized trial. *J. Allergy Clin. Immunol.* **2017**, *140*, 1024–1031.e14. [CrossRef]
75. Tuttle, K.L.; Buchheit, K.M.; Laidlaw, T.M.; Cahill, K.N. A retrospective analysis of mepolizumab in subjects with aspirin-exacerbated respiratory disease. *J. Allergy Clin. Immunol. Pract.* **2018**, *6*, 1045–1047. [CrossRef] [PubMed]

76. Bachert, C.; Mannent, L.; Naclerio, R.M.; Mullol, J.; Ferguson, B.J.; Gevaert, P.; Hellings, P.; Jiao, L.; Wang, L.; Evans, R.R.; et al. Effect of Subcutaneous Dupilumab on Nasal Polyp Burden in Patients With Chronic Sinusitis and Nasal Polyposis: A Randomized Clinical Trial. *JAMA* **2016**, *315*, 469–479. [CrossRef] [PubMed]
77. Wenzel, S.; Castro, M.; Corren, J.; Maspero, J.; Wang, L.; Zhang, B.; Pirozzi, G.; Sutherland, E.R.; Evans, R.R.; Joish, V.N.; et al. Dupilumab efficacy and safety in adults with uncontrolled persistent asthma despite use of medium-to-high-dose inhaled corticosteroids plus a long-acting beta2 agonist: A randomised double-blind placebo-controlled pivotal phase 2b dose-ranging trial. *Lancet* **2016**, *388*, 31–44. [CrossRef]
78. Mullol, J.; Laidlaw, T.M.; Dong, Q. Dupilumab improves nasal polyp burden and asthma control in patients with CRSwNP and NSAID-ERD. *Allergy Asthma Immunol. Res.* **2018**, *73*, 203.
79. McFadden, E.A.; Kany, R.J.; Fink, J.N.; Toohill, R.J. Surgery for sinusitis and aspirin triad. *Laryngoscope* **1990**, *100*, 1043–1046. [CrossRef] [PubMed]
80. Abouali, O.; Keshavarzian, E.; Farhadi, G.; Faramarzi, A.; Ahmadi, G.; Bagheri, M. Micro and nanoparticle deposition in human nasal passage pre and post virtual maxillary sinus endoscopic surgery. *Respir. Physiol. Neurobiol.* **2012**, *181*, 335–345. [CrossRef]
81. Kumar, H.; Jain, R. Review: The role of computational simulation in understanding the postoperative sinonasal environment. *Clin. Biomech.* **2018**. [CrossRef]
82. Jerschow, E.; Edin, M.; Chi, Y.; Hurst, B.; Abuzeid, W.; Akbar, N.; Gibber, M.; Fried, M.; Han, W.; Pelletier, T.; et al. Sinus surgery is associated with a decrease in aspirin-induced reaction severity in AERD patients. *J. Allergy Clin. Immunol. Pract.* **2018**. [CrossRef]
83. Mendelsohn, D.; Jeremic, G.; Wright, E.; Rotenberg, B. Revision rates after endoscopic sinus surgery: A recurrence analysis. *Ann. Otol. Rhinol. Laryngol.* **2011**, *120*, 162–166. [CrossRef]
84. Lee, R.; Stevenson, D. Aspirin-Exacerbated Respiratory Disease: Evaluation and Management. *Allergy Asthma Immunol. Res.* **2011**, *3*, 3–10. [CrossRef]
85. Cho, K.S.; Soudry, E.; Psaltis, A.J.; Nadeau, K.C.; McGhee, S.A.; Nayak, J.V.; Hwang, P.H. Long-term sinonasal outcomes of aspirin desensitization in aspirin exacerbated respiratory disease. *Otolaryngol. Head Neck Surg.* **2014**, *151*, 575–581. [CrossRef]
86. Havel, M.; Ertl, L.; Braunschweig, F.; Markmann, S.; Leunig, A.; Gamarra, F.; Kramer, M.F. Sinonasal outcome under aspirin desensitization following functional endoscopic sinus surgery in patients with aspirin triad. *Eur. Arch. Otorhinolaryngol.* **2013**, *270*, 571–578. [CrossRef] [PubMed]
87. Walters, K.M.; Waldram, J.D.; Woessner, K.M.; White, A.A. Long-term Clinical Outcomes of Aspirin Desensitization With Continuous Daily Aspirin Therapy in Aspirin-exacerbated Respiratory Disease. *Am. J. Rhinol. Allergy* **2018**, *32*, 280–286. [CrossRef] [PubMed]
88. Stevenson, D.D.; Hankammer, M.A.; Mathison, D.A.; Christiansen, S.C.; Simon, R.A. Aspirin desensitization treatment of aspirin-sensitive patients with rhinosinusitis-asthma: Long-term outcomes. *J. Allergy Clin. Immunol.* **1996**, *98*, 751–758. [CrossRef]
89. Adappa, N.D.; Ranasinghe, V.J.; Trope, M.; Brooks, S.G.; Glicksman, J.T.; Parasher, A.K.; Palmer, J.N.; Bosso, J.V. Outcomes after complete endoscopic sinus surgery and aspirin desensitization in aspirin-exacerbated respiratory disease. *Int. Forum Allergy Rhinol.* **2018**, *8*, 49–53. [CrossRef]
90. Stevens, W.; Peters, A.; Hirsch, A.; Nordberg, C.; Schwartz, B.; Mercer, D.; Mahdavinia, M.; Grammer, L.; Hulse, K.; Kern, R.; et al. Clinical Characteristics of Patients with Chronic Rhinosinusitis with Nasal Polyps, Asthma, and Aspirin-Exacerbated Respiratory Disease. *J. Allergy Clin. Immunol. Pract.* **2017**, *5*, 1061–1070. [CrossRef]
91. Morrissey, D.K.; Bassiouni, A.; Psaltis, A.J.; Naidoo, Y.; Wormald, P.J. Outcomes of revision endoscopic modified Lothrop procedure. *Int. Forum Allergy Rhinol.* **2016**, *6*, 518–522. [CrossRef] [PubMed]
92. Ragab, S.M.; Lund, V.J.; Scadding, G. Evaluation of the medical and surgical treatment of chronic rhinosinusitis: A prospective, randomised, controlled trial. *Laryngoscope* **2004**, *114*, 923–930. [CrossRef] [PubMed]
93. Eloy, J.A.; Marchiano, E.; Vazquez, A. Extended Endoscopic and Open Sinus Surgery for Refractory Chronic Rhinosinusitis. *Otolaryngol. Clin. N. Am.* **2017**, *50*, 165–182. [CrossRef] [PubMed]
94. Metson, R.; Sindwani, R. Endoscopic surgery for frontal sinusitis–a graduated approach. *Otolaryngol. Clin. N. Am.* **2004**, *37*, 411–422. [CrossRef]

95. Abuzeid, W.M.; Vakil, M.; Lin, J.; Fastenberg, J.; Akbar, N.A.; Fried, M.P.; Fang, C.H. Endoscopic modified Lothrop procedure after failure of primary endoscopic sinus surgery: A meta-analysis. *Int. Forum Allergy Rhinol.* **2018**, *8*, 605–613. [CrossRef] [PubMed]
96. Naidoo, Y.; Bassiouni, A.; Keen, M.; Wormald, P.J. Long-term outcomes for the endoscopic modified Lothrop/Draf III procedure: A 10-year review. *Laryngoscope* **2014**, *124*, 43–49. [CrossRef] [PubMed]
97. Stammberger, H.; Posawetz, W. Functional endoscopic sinus surgery. Concept, indications and results of the Messerklinger technique. *Eur. Arch. Otorhinolaryngol.* **1990**, *247*, 63–76. [CrossRef]
98. DeConde, A.; Suh, J.; Mace, J.; Alt, J.; Smith, T. Outcomes of complete vs targeted approaches to endoscopic sinus surgery. *Int. Forum Allergy Rhinol.* **2015**, *5*, 691–700. [CrossRef] [PubMed]
99. Abuzeid, W.M.; Mace, J.C.; Costa, M.L.; Rudmik, L.; Soler, Z.M.; Kim, G.S.; Smith, T.L.; Hwang, P.H. Outcomes of chronic frontal sinusitis treated with ethmoidectomy: A prospective study. *Int. Forum Allergy Rhinol.* **2016**, *6*, 597–604. [CrossRef] [PubMed]
100. Eloy, J.A.; Vazquez, A.; Liu, J.K.; Baredes, S. Endoscopic Approaches to the Frontal Sinus: Modifications of the Existing Techniques and Proposed Classification. *Otolaryngol. Clin. N. Am.* **2016**, *49*, 1007–1018. [CrossRef] [PubMed]
101. Zhao, K.; Craig, J.; Cohen, N.; Adappa, N.; Khalili, S.; Palmer, J. Sinus irrigations before and after surgery-Visualization through computational fluid dynamics simulations. *Laryngoscope* **2017**, *126*, E90–E96. [CrossRef]
102. Anderson, P.; Sindwani, R. Safety and efficacy of the endoscopic modified Lothrop procedure: A systematic review and meta-analysis. *Laryngoscope* **2009**, *119*, 1828–1833. [CrossRef]
103. Jankowski, R.; Pigret, D.; Decroocq, F.; Blum, A.; Gillet, P. Comparison of radical (nasalisation) and functional ethmoidectomy in patients with severe sinonasal polyposis. A retrospective study. *Rev. Laryngol. Otol. Rhinol. (Bord)* **2006**, *127*, 131–140.

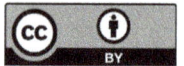

© 2019 by the authors. Licensee MDPI, Basel, Switzerland. This article is an open access article distributed under the terms and conditions of the Creative Commons Attribution (CC BY) license (http://creativecommons.org/licenses/by/4.0/).

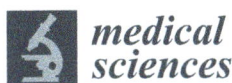

Review

The Role of the Adenoids in Pediatric Chronic Rhinosinusitis

Ryan Belcher and Frank Virgin *

Department of Otolaryngology, Vanderbilt University Medical Center, Vanderbilt University, Nashville, TN 37235, USA; ryan.belcher@vumc.edu
* Correspondence: frank.w.virgin@vumc.org

Received: 21 January 2019; Accepted: 21 February 2019; Published: 25 February 2019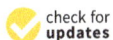

Abstract: There are several mechanisms by which the adenoids contribute to pediatric chronic rhinosinusitis (PCRS), particularly with children aged 12 years and younger. Understanding the role that the adenoids play in PCRS is crucial when attempting to treat these patients. A literature review was performed to address this problem and provide information surrounding this topic. This review will provide a better understanding of how adenoids contribute to PCRS, and also of the medical and surgical treatment options.

Keywords: adenoids; adenoiditis; pediatric; chronic rhinosinusitis; adenoidectomy; sinusitis; biofilm

1. Introduction

Pediatric chronic rhinosinusitis (PCRS) is a condition commonly encountered in otolaryngology practice. Pediatric patients acquire a large burden of upper respiratory tract infections (URTI), with 5–13% of these URTIs progressing to acute bacterial sinusitis, and a proportion of those progressing to PCRS [1]. The disease is diagnosed in 2.1% of children in ambulatory healthcare visits per year in the United States and is known to have a significant impact on health-related quality of life [2]. Due to the increased awareness of the disease's prevalence, over the last eight years multiple professional societies, which include the American Rhinologic Society (ARS) [3], the American Academy of Otolaryngology—Head and Neck Surgery (AAO-HNS) [1], the European Rhinologic Society, and the European Academy of Allergy and Clinical Immunology [4], as well as the Canadian Society of Otolaryngology—Head and Neck Surgery [5], have written clinical consensus statements addressing optimal management of these patients.

There are many factors that contribute to the development of PCRS, including the adenoids, impairment in mucociliary clearance (e.g., primary ciliary dyskinesia, and cystic fibrosis), and anatomic abnormalities of the sinuses, among many others. A major difference between the pathophysiology of the disease process for children compared to adults is the role of the adenoid pad. Adenoids have been shown to have a significant impact on the development of PCRS in children aged 12 years and younger [1,6].

Medical management is considered the first line of therapy in the treatment of PCRS, with surgical intervention reserved for patients who fail to improve with these conservative measures [1]. Due to the understanding of the role the adenoid pad plays in PCRS, adenoidectomy with or without maxillary irrigation is the most commonly performed surgical intervention reported among members of ARS and the American Society of Pediatric Otolaryngology (ASPO) [7,8]. However, evidence has not shown a role for adenoidectomy in pediatric patients 13 years or older [1,9].

Several studies have been performed to evaluate the relationship between the adenoid pad and paranasal sinus in pediatric patients with chronic rhinosinusitis (CRS), and this review looks to summarize these studies, specifically looking at disease presentation, adenoiditis, obstruction, biofilm formation, colonization, immune function, and medical and surgical management.

2. Disease Presentation/Diagnosis

Pediatric chronic rhinosinusitis is defined as at least 90 continuous days of symptoms of purulent rhinorrhea, nasal obstruction, facial pressure/pain, or a cough with corresponding endoscopic and/or computed tomography (CT) findings in a patient who is 18 years of age or younger [1]. Thus obtaining a thorough and complete history and physical is important for establishing a diagnosis. It is important to note that age is a distinguishing factor in the diagnosis of PCRS in that allergic rhinitis is a more prominent factor in older children, whereas adenoid disease (independent of adenoid size) is a more important contributing factor in younger children [1].

As the PCRS definition states, CT is the gold standard for imaging when establishing a PCRS diagnosis or preparing for sinus surgery, particularly a non-contrasted CT with axial, coronal, and sagittal views. The sensitivity and specificity of plain radiographs, such as a lateral soft tissue neck X-ray evaluating the adenoids, are limited in evaluating the patient's need for adenoidectomy [10,11]. According to the AAO-HNS consensus on appropriate use of CT imaging, it is recommended in patients with PCRS when medical management and/or adenoidectomy have failed to control symptoms [11]. Practice patterns differentiate between otolaryngologists on whether to obtain CT imaging before adenoidectomy with 82% of surveyed ASPO members elected to perform adenoidectomy prior to obtaining a CT scan compared to 40% of surveyed ARS members ($p < 0.001$) [7,8]. Bhattacharyya et al., in 2004, showed that a CT with a Lund-Mackay score of ≥ 5 had good sensitivity and specificity in establishing a diagnosis of PCRS in children not responsive to medical treatment [12].

Nasal endoscopy is another option in the armamentarium of otolaryngologists in the evaluation of PCRS. While nasal endoscopy can be useful in the diagnosis of PCRS, it can also be used to diagnose adenoiditis and adenoid hyperplasia. In a survey of otolaryngologists, 48% reported that they always or almost always use nasal endoscopy to establish a diagnosis of PCRS, with 21% reporting usually, and 26% sometimes [8].

3. Pathophysiology of Adenoid Contribution to Pediatric Chronic Rhinosinusitis

Adenoid tissue is implicated in contributing to PCRS by several different mechanisms, which include serving as a bacterial reservoir and causing posterior nasal obstruction [13]. Both of these are thought to be factors in causing impaired mucociliary clearance of the sinus cavities. Similar to the sinus mucosa, the adenoids are lined by a layer of ciliated epithelium that can undergo metaplastic change and loss of cilia as a consequence of recurrent or chronic inflammation [13,14]. Posterior nasal obstruction can cause mucous retention in the sinus cavity and in the adenoid pad, which in turn can cause microbial colonization and subsequent inflammation of the mucosa. When an adenoidectomy is performed in this context it relieves the posterior nasal obstruction and removes a significant bacterial reservoir, allowing for better clearance of nasal secretions. Decreased nasal mucosal inflammation can result in improved mucociliary clearance and lead to less sinus ostial obstruction from mucosal edema and better sinus ventilation and drainage [13]. In an attempt to prove this concept, Arnaoutakis et al. used Andersen's saccharine test in 10 patients with adenoid hypertrophy, chronic adenoiditis, or PCRS to measure the nasal mucociliary clearance time (MCT) and mucociliary velocity (MCV) before and after adenoidectomy. They found that both MCT and MCV improved postoperatively among the group, which was considered to be clinically relevant. However, the small population size precluded testing for statistical significance [13].

Bacterial biofilms have been shown to cover tonsillar, adenoid, and sinus mucosa. In comparing PCRS patients vs. obstructive sleep apnea (control) patients receiving adenoidectomy, Zuliani et al. demonstrated identifiable biofilms covering almost the entire mucosal surface on all adenoid specimens from PCRS patients and no biofilms from the obstructive sleep apnea patients [15]. Biofilms can be problematic due to their decreased metabolic activity and expression and transmission of resistance genes. These characteristics may lead to decreased or incomplete penetration of antimicrobials as well as unique antimicrobial resistance patterns [15]. This can also allow sinus microbials to persist in the nasopharynx in PCRS, resulting in minimal to no improvement after frequent antibiotic courses administered. Not surprisingly, biofilms themselves have been shown to cause a state of chronic inflammation to the surrounding tissue that may not even be involved in the microbial infections [15]. The most common pathogenic organisms identified in the adenoids include *Staphylococcus aureus*, *Streptococcus pneumoniae*, *Haemophilus influenzae*, and group A *streptococci* [16]. These same bacteria are similar to the common organisms found in acute and chronic sinusitis in children [17]. The presence of biofilms on adenoid tissue in PCRS is another example that supports the role of an adenoidectomy in that it mechanically removes a potential nidus for re-infection of the sinuses.

The adenoids are covered in respiratory epithelium and are therefore considered in part a secretory immunological organ that provides local secretory immunoglobulin A (IgA) that contributes directly to regional surface protection. Immunoglobulin A is an important immunoglobulin in the upper respiratory tract as it binds to bacteria and suppresses colonization. When compared to controls, Eun et al. found that adenoid tissue in patients with otitis media (OM) and PCRS had a significantly lower amount of IgA ($p = 0.016$ and $p = 0.004$, respectively). They postulate that the increased susceptibility to infection in these patients was likely caused by the reduction in IgA [18]. Further research in the immunological side of PCRS and adenoids is needed to elucidate whether the decreased IgA is caused by concomitant inflammation or if these patients are innately deficient in IgA in their upper respiratory tract, making them more susceptible to chronic inflammation and subsequent PCRS.

Even though posterior nasal obstruction is thought to contribute to PCRS, no studies have been able to correlate the size of the adenoid pad with the presence of sinonasal symptoms in PCRS. No association has been found, whether the studies have looked at radiographic evidence of nasopharyngeal obstruction by adenoid hypertrophy [19], at the volume [20], or at the weight of adenoid tissue removed [21]. Another potential causative agent that has been investigated for adenoiditis and/or PCRS is *Helicobacter pylori*. The majority of studies evaluating this relationship have been performed in the adult population; however, there are an increasing number of studies being performed in the pediatric population as more non-invasive techniques for detecting *H. pylori* have been developed. In the pediatric studies, regardless of technique, no studies have consistently been able to identify *H. pylori* or structures compatible with the microorganism with most studies finding no evidence of bacteria in their samples [22]. Recently, Grateron Cedeno et al. failed to detect the presence of *H. pylori* in adenoid tissue or maxillary sinus in PCRS patients despite using high-sensitivity and -specificity diagnostic techniques. In their conclusion they emphasize an unlikely role of the microorganism in PCRS without nasal polyps and adenoidal hypertrophy and/or chronic adenoiditis etiology [22].

4. Treatment

Whether the adenoids are implicated or not, medical management is considered the first line of therapy in the treatment of PCRS. The duration and combination of medications that constitute "maximal medical therapy" is still under debate. Studies have shown that a topical nasal steroid spray and daily, topical nasal irrigations are beneficial medical therapies [1]. Once-daily nasal saline irrigations have been shown to improve quality of life and Lund-Mackay scores after just six weeks in PCRS [23]. The use of antimicrobials in the treatment of PCRS is known to be widespread, with no agreed-upon optimal duration. The AAO-HNS consensus statement reports that 20 days of antibiotic therapy may produce a superior response in PCRS patients compared to 10 days of antibiotics. However, the panel failed to reach consensus on the appropriate antibiotic duration in PCRS, but stated that it should be a minimum of 10 consecutive days [1]. It was also agreed upon that culture-directed antibiotics may improve outcomes when patients have not responded to empirical antibiotic treatment [1].

A survey of ASPO members evaluated their members' preferences when it comes to maximal medical therapy. One hundred fifteen members responded to the survey. Within this response group, the most common medications used within their "maximal medical" therapy were nasal steroid sprays (96%), saline irrigations (93%), and oral antibiotics (91%) [7]. Less commonly included medications in their regimens were oral steroids (43%), oral antihistamines (38%), anti-leukotrienes (36%), anti-reflux medications (26%), nasal antihistamine sprays (20%), nasal steroid irrigations (19%), nebulized antibiotics or steroids (7%), and intravenous antibiotics (3%) [7]. When it came to utilizing antibiotics, 65% treat for 15–21 days, 24% treat for >21 days, and 11% for <14 days [7]. Of note, this ASPO survey was completed two years after the AAO-HNS PCRS clinical consensus statement was published.

5. Surgical Treatment

Surgical intervention is reserved for patients with PCRS that have failed "maximal medical therapy." There are several options for surgery in these patients including adenoidectomy and endoscopic sinus surgery (ESS), which have an age- and anatomy-dependent differentiation. Given the role that the adenoids have been shown to play in the etiology of PCRS for children 12 years and younger, adenoidectomy should be considered as a first-line surgical option [1]. It is a simple, well-tolerated procedure and a meta-analysis evaluating the efficacy of adenoidectomy alone in the PCRS population demonstrated a success rate of approximately 70%, in which patients had improved sinusitis symptoms after intervention [24]. Although the tonsils are a part of Waldeyer's ring and have similar bacteriology, tonsillectomy is considered an ineffective treatment for PCRS [1]. Ramadan et al. showed that children with chronic adenoiditis, which has similar symptoms to PCRS, who had a CT scan with a Lund-Mackay score of ≤ 5 and received an adenoidectomy had a higher success rate than children with chronic adenoiditis and CRS (65% versus 43%; $p = 0.0017$) [25]. This study also showed that asthmatic children with CRS had a very poor response rate to adenoidectomy alone when compared with asthmatic children with CA (28% versus 53%; $p = 0.022$) [25].

Adjunctive procedures can also be performed at the same time as the adenoidectomy; most commonly, these are maxillary sinus irrigations or balloon sinuplasty. Ramadan et al. showed that adenoidectomy with the addition of maxillary sinus irrigation in PCRS resulted in improved one-year outcomes (87.5%) vs. adenoidectomy alone (60.7%) [26]. Since the U.S. Food and Drug Administration approved balloon catheter sinuplasty in 2006 it has emerged as a potential treatment option for PCRS. Several studies have evaluated the role of balloon sinuplasty in PCRS. Ramadan et al. [27] performed balloon sinuplasty alone versus adenoidectomy in a group of PCRS patients. This study demonstrated superior improvement in symptoms at one year in the balloon group (80%) vs. adenoidectomy group (52.6%) [28]. A more recent randomized, blinded study that evaluated the impact of adding balloon catheter dilation to adenoidectomy with maxillary irrigation did not demonstrate any improved benefit at one year [6].

In patients in which PCRS is persistent despite adenoidectomy, the otolaryngologist can then consider performing an ESS. There is a lack of convincing evidence at this time that ESS causes a clinically significant impairment of facial growth in children with CRS, so may be appropriate at any age [1]. In order to optimize the outcomes of all treatments or interventions, appropriately treating concomitant issues such as asthma has been shown to improve the outcomes of PCRS. Accordingly, there is evidence that clinical control of PCRS is important in aiding in the control of asthma [29]. Other factors or underlying diagnoses that may lead to persistent or recalcitrant PCRS despite interventions should be considered and investigated further, such as cystic fibrosis, allergies, primary ciliary dyskinesia, and immunodeficiencies.

6. Conclusions

The adenoid pad plays a key role in the etiology of PCRS through several mechanisms, particularly for children aged 12 and younger. Should these PCRS patients fail maximal medical therapy, adenoidectomy +/− adjunctive treatments should be considered first-line surgical intervention.

Author Contributions: Conceptualization, R.B. and F.V.; Methodology; R.B and F.V.; Writing-Original Draft Preparation, R.B.; Writing-Review & Editing, R.B. and F.V.; Visualization, R.B. and F.V.; Supervision, F.V.

Conflicts of Interest: The authors declare no conflict of interest.

References

1. Brietzke, S.E.; Shin, J.J.; Choi, S.; Lee, J.T.; Parikh, S.R.; Pena, M.; Prager, J.D.; Ramadan, H.; Veling, M.; Corrigan, M.; et al. Clinical consensus statement: Pediatric chronic rhinosinusitis. *Otolaryngol. Head Neck Surg.* **2014**, *151*, 542–553. [CrossRef] [PubMed]
2. Gilani, S.; Shin, J.J. The burden and visit prevalence of pediatric chronic rhinosinusitis. *Otolaryngol. Head Neck Surg.* **2017**, *157*, 1048–1052. [CrossRef] [PubMed]
3. Orlandi, R.R.; Kingdom, T.T.; Hwang, P.H.; Smith, T.L.; Alt, J.A.; Baroody, F.M.; Batra, P.S.; Bernal-Sprekelsen, M.; Bhattacharyya, N.; Chandra, R.K.; et al. International consensus statement on allergy and rhinology: Rhinosinusitis. *Int. Forum Allergy Rhinol.* **2016**, *6* (Suppl. S1), S22–S209. [CrossRef] [PubMed]
4. Fokkens, W.J.; Lund, V.J.; Mullol, J.; Bachert, C.; Alobid, I.; Baroody, F.; Cohen, N.; Cervin, A.; Douglas, R.; Gevaert, P.; et al. EPOS 2012: European position paper on rhinosinusitis and nasal polyps 2012. A summary for otorhinolaryngologists. *Rhinology* **2012**, *50*, 1–12. [CrossRef] [PubMed]
5. Desrosiers, M.; Evans, G.A.; Keith, P.K.; Wright, E.D.; Kaplan, A.; Bouchard, J.; Ciavarella, A.; Doyle, P.W.; Javer, A.R.; Leith, E.S.; et al. Canadian clinical practice guidelines for acute and chronic rhinosinusitis. *J. Otolaryngol. Head Neck Surg.* **2011**, *40* (Suppl. S2), S99–S193. [CrossRef] [PubMed]
6. Gerber, M.E.; Kennedy, A.A. Adenoidectomy with balloon catheter sinuplasty: A randomized trial for pediatric rhinosinusitis. *Laryngoscope* **2018**, *128*, 2893–2897. [CrossRef] [PubMed]
7. Beswick, D.M.; Messner, A.H.; Hwang, P.H. Pediatric chronic rhinosinusitis management in rhinologist and pediatric otolaryngologists. *Ann. Otol. Rhinol. Laryngol.* **2017**, *126*, 634–639. [CrossRef] [PubMed]
8. Beswick, D.M.; Ramadan, H.; Baroody, F.; Hwang, P.H. Practice patterns in pediatric chronic rhinosinusitis: A survey of the American Rhinologic Society. *Am. J. Rhinol. Allergy* **2016**, *30*, 418–423. [CrossRef] [PubMed]
9. Neff, L.; Adil, E.A. What is the role of the adenoid in pediatric chronic rhinosinusitis? *Laryngoscope* **2015**, *125*, 1282–1283. [CrossRef] [PubMed]
10. Heath, J.; Hartzell, L.; Putt, C.; Kennedy, J.L. Chronic rhinosinusitis in children: Pathophysiology, evaluation, and medical management. *Pediatr. Allergy Immunol.* **2018**, *18*, 37. [CrossRef] [PubMed]
11. Setzen, G.; Ferguson, B.J.; Han, J.K.; Rhee, J.S.; Cornelius, R.S.; Froum, S.J.; Gillman, G.S.; Houser, S.M.; Krakovitz, P.R.; Monfared, A.; et al. Clinical consensus statement: Appropriate use of computed tomography for paranasal sinus disease. *Otolaryngol. Head Neck Surg.* **2012**, *147*, 808–816. [CrossRef] [PubMed]
12. Bhattacharyya, N.; Jones, D.T.; Hill, M.; Shapiro, N.L. The diagnostic accuracy of computed tomography in pediatric chronic rhinosinusitis. *Arch. Otolaryngol. Head Neck Surg.* **2004**, *130*, 1029–1032. [CrossRef] [PubMed]
13. Arnaoutakis, D.; Collins, W.O. Correlation of mucociliary clearance and symptomatology before and after adenoidectomy in children. *Int. J. Pediatr. Otorhinolaryngol.* **2011**, *75*, 1318–1321. [CrossRef] [PubMed]
14. Maurizi, M.; Ottaviani, G.; Paludetti, G.; Almadori, G.; Zappone, C. Adenoid hypertrophy and nasal mucociliary clearance in children. A morphological and functional study. *Int. J. Pediatr. Otorhinolaryngol.* **1984**, *8*, 31–41. [CrossRef]
15. Zuliani, G.; Carron, M.; Gurrola, J.; Coleman, C.; Haupert, M.; Berk, R.; Coticchia, J. Identification of adenoid biofilms in chronic rhinosinusitis. *Int. J. Pediatr. Otorhinolaryngol.* **2006**, *70*, 1613–1617. [CrossRef] [PubMed]
16. Elwany, S.; El-Dine, A.N.; El-Medany, A.; Omran, A.; Mandour, Z.; Abd El-Salam, A. Relationship between bacteriology of the adenoid core and middle meatus in children with sinusitis. *J. Laryngol. Otol.* **2011**, *125*, 279–281. [CrossRef] [PubMed]

17. Orobello, P.W., Jr.; Park, R.I.; Belcher, L.J.; Eggleston, P.; Lederman, H.M.; Banks, J.R.; Modlin, J.F.; Naclerio, R.M. Microbiology of chronic sinusitis in children. *Arch. Otolaryngol. Head Neck Surg.* **1991**, *117*, 980–983. [CrossRef] [PubMed]
18. Eun, Y.G.; Park, D.C.; Kim, S.G.; Kim, M.G.; Yeo, S.G. Immunoglobulins and transcription factors in adenoids of children with otitis media with effusion and chronic rhinosinusitis. *Int. J. Pediatr. Otorhinolaryngol.* **2009**, *73*, 1412–1416. [CrossRef] [PubMed]
19. Shin, K.S.; Cho, S.H.; Kim, K.R.; Tae, K.; Lee, S.H.; Park, C.W.; Jeong, J.H. The role of adenoids in pediatric rhinosinusitis. *Int. J. Pediatr. Otorhinolaryngol.* **2008**, *72*, 1643–1650. [CrossRef] [PubMed]
20. Bercin, A.S.; Ural, A.; Kutluhan, V.; Yurttas, V. Relationship between sinusitis and adenoid size in pediatric age group. *Ann. Otol. Rhinol. Laryngol.* **2007**, *116*, 550–553. [CrossRef] [PubMed]
21. Lee, D.; Rosenfeld, R.M. Adenoid bacteriology and sinonasal symptoms in children. *Otolaryngol. Head Neck Surg.* **1997**, *116*, 301–307. [CrossRef]
22. Grateron Cedeno, E.E.; Ortiz-Princz, D.; Ceballos Figueredo, S.A.; Cavazza Porro, M.E. Adenoid hypertrophy and chronic rhinosinusisits: Helicobacter pylori on antral lavages, adenoid tissue and salival immunoglobuline A on paediatric patients. *Int. J. Pediatr. Otorhinolaryngol.* **2016**, *80*, 82–87. [CrossRef] [PubMed]
23. Wei, J.L.; Sykes, K.J.; Johnson, P.; He, J.; Mayo, M.S. Safety and efficacy of once-daily nasal irrigation for the treatment of pediatric chronic rhinosinusitis. *Laryngoscope* **2011**, *121*, 1989–2000. [CrossRef] [PubMed]
24. Brietzke, S.E.; Brigger, M.T. Adenoidectomy outcomes in pediatric rhinosinusitis: A meta-analysis. *Int. J. Pediatr. Otorhinolaryngol.* **2008**, *72*, 1541–1545. [CrossRef] [PubMed]
25. Ramadan, H.H.; Makary, C.A. Can computed tomography score predict outcome of adenoidectomy for chronic rhinosinusitis in children. *Am. J. Rhinol. Allergy* **2014**, *28*, e80–e82. [CrossRef] [PubMed]
26. Ramadan, H.H.; Cost, J.L. Outcome of adenoidectomy versus adenoidectomy with maxillary sinus wash for chronic rhinosinusitis in children. *Laryngoscope* **2008**, *118*, 871–873. [CrossRef] [PubMed]
27. Ramadan, H.H.; Terrell, A.M. Balloon catheter sinuplasty and adenoidectomy in children with chronic rhinosinusitis. *Ann. Otol. Laryngol. Rhinol.* **2010**, *119*, 578–582. [CrossRef]
28. Soler, Z.M.; Rosenbloom, J.S.; Skarada, D.; Gutman, M.; Hoy, M.J.; Nguyen, S.A. Prospective multicenter evaluation of balloon sinus dilation for treatment of pediatric chronic rhinosinusitis. *Int. Forum Allergy Rhinol.* **2017**, *7*, 221–229. [CrossRef] [PubMed]
29. Karatzanis, A.; Kalogjera, L.; Scadding, G.; Velegrakis, S.; Kawauchi, H.; Cingi, C.; Prokopakis, E. Severe chronic upper airway disease (SCUAD) in children. Definition issues and requirements. *Int. J. Pediatr. Otorhinolaryngol.* **2015**, *79*, 965–968. [CrossRef] [PubMed]

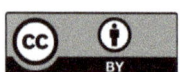

© 2019 by the authors. Licensee MDPI, Basel, Switzerland. This article is an open access article distributed under the terms and conditions of the Creative Commons Attribution (CC BY) license (http://creativecommons.org/licenses/by/4.0/).

Review

Chronic Rhinosinusitis in Cystic Fibrosis: Diagnosis and Medical Management

Chetan Safi [1], Zhong Zheng [1], Emily Dimango [2], Claire Keating [2] and David A. Gudis [1,*]

1. Department of Otolaryngology—Head and Neck Surgery, Columbia University Irving Medical Center; New York, NY 10032, USA; chetansafi@gmail.com (C.S.); zz2618@cumc.columbia.edu (Z.Z.)
2. Department of Pulmonary, Allergy, and Critical Care Medicine, Columbia University Irving Medical Center; New York, NY 10032, USA; ead3@cumc.columbia.edu (E.D.); ck2132@cumc.columbia.edu (C.K.)
* Correspondence: dag62@cumc.columbia.edu; Tel.: +212-305-8555

Received: 20 January 2019; Accepted: 18 February 2019; Published: 22 February 2019

Abstract: Chronic rhinosinusitis (CRS) is nearly ubiquitous in patients with cystic fibrosis (CF). CF CRS is a challenging entity to define, diagnose, and treat, as patients often have severe refractory sinus disease in addition to complex medical comorbidities. The purpose of this article is to review the literature on the medical management of CF CRS and determine how to best identify, diagnose, and manage CF CRS. Ultimately, the treatment of these patients requires a multi-disciplinary approach involving the pulmonologist and otolaryngologist.

Keywords: rhinosinusitis; cystic fibrosis; diagnosis; medical management

1. Introduction

Cystic fibrosis (CF) is an autosomal recessive genetic disorder characterized by poor chloride ion (Cl⁻) transport across cell membranes due to mutations in the cystic fibrosis transmembrane conductance (*CFTR*) gene. It is a systemic disease that can affect the sinopulmonary, gastrointestinal, and genitourinary systems [1]. Reduced chloride transport leads to reduced water crossing the epithelium into mucosal secretions, resulting in thick, inspissated mucus. The pulmonary morbidity of CF is due to this thickened mucus that results in poor mucociliary clearance, secondary bacterial colonization, and recurrent infectious exacerbations that ultimately decrease overall lung function [2]. This continuous process of mucosal inflammation and infection can also affect the paranasal sinuses, leading to chronic rhinosinusitis [3]. Moreover, in considering a unified airway model, some investigators have demonstrated that in CF patients, the paranasal sinuses can serve as a reservoir for virulent bacteria that can then lead to pulmonary exacerbations [4–6]. Thus, collaboration with a CF pulmonologist is essential to diagnose and treat chronic rhinosinusitis in these complex patients. In this review, our aim is to identify the best strategies to diagnose cystic fibrosis chronic rhinosinusitis (CF CRS) as well as review the medical therapies available to treat these patients. The indications and benefits of surgical therapy are outside the scope of this review.

2. Diagnosis

One challenge in treating CF CRS is defining the disease and identifying patients. The International Consensus Statement on Allergy and Rhinology states that CRS is defined by persistent sinus inflammation for over 12 weeks with the presence of subjective symptoms and objective measures [7]. Subjective symptoms include nasal obstruction, purulent rhinorrhea, facial pain or pressure, and hyposmia or anosmia. Objective findings include purulent sinonasal discharge, mucosal edema, or nasal polyps on nasal endoscopy with evidence of mucosal inflammation on cross-sectional imaging [7]. However, unlike in patients without CF, there is often not a correlation between symptoms and objective measures of sinonasal disease in CF patients. While 60–80% of CF patients have radiographic evidence of CRS, fewer than 20% of patients will spontaneously report symptoms [3,8]. Nevertheless, physicians today still use quality of life metrics, nasal endoscopy, and cross-sectional imaging to assess patients for CF CRS.

3. Quality of Life Metrics

CRS symptoms of nasal obstruction, purulent rhinorrhea, facial pain, and hyposmia, can have a dramatic impact on some patients' quality of life (QOL). Hopkins et al. showed that the Sinonasal Outcome Test-22 (SNOT-22) is a validated instrument that includes rhinologic, extra-nasal rhinologic, aural/facial, psychologic dysfunction, and sleep dysfunction domains that can be used to determine the effect of CRS on a patient's QOL as well as assess the outcome of surgical therapy [9]. Habib et al. compared CF patients with and without CRS and found that a SNOT-22 score greater than 21 was indicative of concomitant CRS in CF patients [10]. Moreover, the study found that SNOT-22, as a single variable predictor, did not differ from a multivariable regression model, including several sociodemographic and clinical variables, in determining the presence or absence of CRS [10]. Another study found that the respiratory component of the Cystic Fibrosis Questionnaire—Revised for adults and adolescents above age 14, a CF-specific QOL metric, was statistically lower in patients with CRS compared to patients without CRS. This indicates worsened perceived respiratory health in patients with chronic sinus disease [11].

Another QOL instrument studied in the pediatric CF population is the Sinus and Nasal Quality of Life Survey (SN-5). The SN-5 has been validated as a reliable health-related QOL survey in children ages two to fourteen with sinonasal symptoms [12]. It asks parents about their child's sinus infections, nasal obstruction, allergy symptoms, emotional distress, and activity limitations [12]. Wentzell et al. found that SN-5 scores significantly correlated with recent episodes of sinusitis, antibiotic prescriptions for sinusitis, and number of days missed from school, concluding that this instrument is a reliable method for monitoring sinonasal symptoms in children with CF [13]. Xie et al. found that all 5 domains of the SN-5 correlated with a change in overall QOL scores for children aged zero to four; however, for children aged five to twelve and thirteen to eighteen only two or less subdomains of the SN-5 correlated with overall QOL. They suggested that an overall better instrument be developed to evaluate older children and adolescent CF patients with CRS [14].

4. Nasal Endoscopy/Computed Tomography

Nasal endoscopy is another tool commonly used by otolaryngologists in diagnosing paranasal sinus pathology. For CF patients with sinonasal disease, nasal endoscopy can reveal thick nasal drainage, mucosal edema, and nasal polyposis [4,8,15]. However, these findings can be non-specific and do not always correlate with symptoms [15]. Casserly et al. demonstrated that CF patients with and without subjective symptoms of sinus disease had similar Lund–Kennedy nasal endoscopy (LKNE) scores which were overall worse than the general population without CRS. These findings indicate that the inflammatory component of CF can produce a clinically detectable difference in sinus and nasal mucosal health on nasal endoscopy. However, the challenge with CF patients is reconciling this objective data with subjective symptomatology when considering medical or surgical intervention.

Computed tomography without contrast is indispensable in evaluating patients for CF CRS. Common findings include sphenoid or frontal hypoplasia/aplasia, medial bulging of the lateral nasal wall, demineralization of the uncinate process, sphenoethmoidal recess inflammation, sinus opacification, osteitis and neogenesis, and sclerosis of paranasal sinus bone [16–18]. However, as with nasal endoscopy, there is evidence that CT findings do not always correlate with symptoms. Kang et al. found that while 84.7% of their CF cohort had radiologic evidence of CRS, there was no statistically significant difference in Lund-MacKay scores amongst patients stratified based on the severity of their sinonasal symptoms on SNOT-22 [16]. They question whether this dichotomy between imaging and symptoms is a sign of true lack of pathologic inflammation or simply an underreporting of symptoms in the presence of real sinus disease [16]. Furthermore, Rasmussen et al. states that cross-sectional imaging with CT should not be the single determinant when considering ESS as there is no correlation between imaging findings and detection of pus or pathogenic bacteria [19]. Purulence and pathogenic bacteria were found in patients without sinus opacification on CT and sterile cultures were also found in patients with sinus opacification [19]. Due to these imaging uncertainties, some have developed a novel CT scoring system which combines characteristics such as lateral nasal wall bulging and sinus opacification with uncinate demineralization and mucocele presence to quantify severity of sinus disease in CF patients [20]. With respect to children with CF, authors have shown that most patients between 0 and 17 years old will have more severe sinus opacification than their non-CF counterparts [17]. Thus, to limit excessive radiation, CT scans should only be used for peri-operative evaluation and for assessment of sinusitis-related complications [21].

The relationship between CF patients' genotype and resultant severity of sinus disease has also been assessed. Abuzeid et al. found that patients with high risk CF genotypes, such as class I–III mutations which lead to markedly diminished presence or activity of the cystic fibrosis transmembrane regulator chloride channel, have no statistically significant difference in their SNOT-22, Lund–Mackay, and LKNE scores when compared to low-risk CF genotypes, such as class IV–V mutations, after controlling for confounding variables [22]. The class of mutations are determined based on the mechanism of how they disrupt the *CFTR* gene with categories ranging from defective synthesis of *CFTR* in class I mutations to reduced synthesis or stability of active *CFTR* in class V mutations [22]. On the other hand, Berkhout et al. evaluated CT scans in CF patients and found that those with class I–III mutations had a statistically higher Lund–Mackay score per component of sinonasal system when compared to patients with class IV–V mutations [8]. They noted significantly smaller frontal and sphenoid sinuses, more overall paranasal sinus opacification, and more osteitis/neoosteogenesis of the maxillary sinus wall in the high risk genotype group [8].

Based on the above findings, both nasal endoscopy and computed tomography should be used concurrently to identify objective characteristics of sinonasal disease in CF patients presenting with sinonasal symptoms. The symptomatic patient with evidence of nasal polyposis, sinonasal mucopurulence, and mucosal edema on nasal endoscopy as well sclerotic bone and opacified paranasal sinuses on CT should possibly be treated for CRS.

5. Treatment

In treating CF-related sinonasal disease, a number of systemic and topical medical therapies have been identified, with varied data supporting their efficacy as seen in Table 1. Dornase-alfa is a mucolytic agent that functions by cleaving extracellular DNA in the airways and improving mucus viscosity while improving lung function and reducing pulmonary exacerbations [23]. In a randomized controlled trial, CF patients underwent nasal nebulized treatment with dornase-alfa or placebo for 1 year after endoscopic sinus surgery [24]. At 48 weeks after surgery, patients receiving dornase alfa had a statistically significant improvement in their sinonasal symptoms, LKNE score, Lund–Mackay score, and forced expiratory volume in 1 s (FEV1) compared with those receiving placebo [24]. When compared to isotonic nasal saline, Mainz et al. found that CF patients treated with nebulized intranasal dornase-alfa had statistically significant improvement in SNOT-22 scores as well as in forced expiratory flow 75–25% [25].

Nasal saline irrigations are also commonly used to treat chronic sinusitis. Mainz et al. performed a randomized controlled trial in which CF patients used both 28 days of isotonic saline irrigations and 28 days of hypertonic (6.0%) saline irrigations with a washout period in-between [26]. In total, 4 mL of saline was administered daily using a nebulizer and was aerosolized into the nasal cavities. Both therapies led to similarly small improvements in SNOT-22 scores, though it is important to consider that hypertonic saline can lead to more irritated mucosa [3,26]. Others have postulated that saline irrigations themselves can be a poor method to clear sinuses of mucus and crusting or to serve as a delivery method for medications such as antibiotics and steroids because of poor sinus penetration. Aanaes et al. found that even after endoscopic sinus surgery, no saline irrigation reached the frontal and sphenoid sinuses as measured by single-photon emission computed tomography, with less than 50% of maxillary sinuses showing an improvement in post-operative sinus fluid volume after irrigation [27].

Topical corticosteroids are another option available in treating CF sinonasal disease. Hadfield et al. performed a randomized controlled trial in which CF patients with nasal polyps were given 6 weeks of either twice daily topical betamethasone or placebo [28]. After six weeks, there was a statistically significant reduction in nasal polyposis but no change in symptom score [28]. In a retrospective series, Donaldson et al. found that 62.5% of CF patients with nasal polyposis had resolution of polyps or smaller polyps after twice daily nasal inhalations of beclomethasone (100 mg) [29]. In the same study, he found that 78.6% of CF patients without nasal polyposis had improvement in nasal obstructive symptoms with the same regimen [29]. Additionally, other authors have demonstrated the efficacy of beclomethasone with respect to nasal polyp size and improved sinus symptomatology [30,31]. However, there is no conclusive data on the use of oral steroids in the CF population when used to manage sinus disease [3]. In terms of safety profile, topical inhaled corticosteroids such as budesonide can be used without causing dysfunction to the hypothalamic-pituitary axis while use of oral corticosteroids should be guarded due to a high incidence of diabetes secondary to pancreatic insufficiency and metabolic disorders in the CF population [3,32,33].

As chronic infection in the upper and lower airways with *Pseudomonas aeruginosa* and *Staphylococcus aureus* are common in CF patients, topical antibiotics are yet another therapy for treating CF-related sinus disease [34]. One study found that after endoscopic sinus surgery, a postoperative regimen of two weeks of broad spectrum intravenous antibiotics, six months of colistin irrigations, and at least 6 months of topical nasal steroids resulted in a negative sinus culture for at least 6 months in about 50 percent of patients [35]. However, it is difficult to determine what degree of reduced colonization can be attributed to surgical versus medical therapy alone. Additionally, in a randomized controlled trial, Mainz et al. found that topical aerosolized tobramycin resulted in a decrease in burden of paranasal sinus *P. aeruginosa* growth as well as a statistically significant improvement in SNOT-20 scores when compared to a placebo [36]. Yet another study found that the re-operation rate for CF patients who underwent serial sinus lavage of antibiotics such as tobramycin after endoscopic sinus surgery versus patients who underwent conventional surgery alone was 10% vs. 47% 1 year postoperatively and 22% vs. 72% 2 years postoperatively, respectively [37]. This evidence suggests that topical antibiotics can be useful in the treatment of CF CRS.

Ivacaftor is a recently developed novel therapy which works as a *CFTR* modulator that acts by restoring *CFTR* ion transport function at the cellular level in patients with specific *CFTR* mutations known as gating mutations [38]. In CF patients with gating mutations, ivacaftor substantially improved baseline lung function, lowered sweat chloride levels to below disease levels, and has slowed deterioration in lung function by nearly fifty percent per year [39,40]. With regards to sinus disease, Chang et al. describes a patient with medically and surgically recalcitrant CF-related sinus disease who developed newly cleared maxillary and frontal sinuses, improved symptomatology, and improved FEV1 after 10 months of ivacaftor therapy [38]. Additionally, in vitro studies also showed evidence of increased ion transport as well as improved viscosity of secretions with ivacaftor [38]. Furthermore, McCormick et al. demonstrated that ivacaftor therapy improved patients' rhinologic, sleep, and psychological domain scores on the SNOT-20 quality of life metric 1 and 3 months after starting therapy, though it should be mentioned that 75% of patients started with a score of <1 on SNOT-20 [41]. There has since been approval of two additional *CFTR* modulator therapies approved for an ever expanding list of *CFTR* genotypes. Though a surplus of data on the modulators' effect on CF CRS is still lacking, it is possible that these groundbreaking drugs, with their ability to restore chloride transport to improve mucociliary clearance in CF, will modify the course and attenuate the severity of disease of the upper airway as it does in the lower airways.

Table 1. Summary of medical management used to treat cystic fibrosis rhinosinusitis.

Reference	Therapeutic	Duration	Outcome
Cimmino et al. [24]	Dornase-alpha	48 weeks	Improved sinonasal symptoms, LKNE score, LMS, and FEV1
Mainz et al. [25]	Dornase-alpha	4 weeks	Improved SNOT-22 and forced expiratory flow 75%–25%
Mainz et al. [26]	Isotonic vs. hypertonic saline	4 weeks	Both led to similar small improvements in SNOT-22
Hadfield et al. [28]	Beclomethasone	6 weeks	Reduction in polyposis but no change in symptom score
Donaldson et al. [29]	Beclomethasone	Not described	Improvement in nasal polyposis and nasal obstruction
Aanaes et al. [35]	Colistin irrigations	6 months	Negative sinus cultures for at least 6 months in at least 50% of patients
Mainz et al. [36]	Nebulized tobramycin	4 weeks–8 weeks	Decreased burden of *P. aeruginosa* and improvement in SNOT-22
Moss et al. [37]	Tobramycin lavage	7–10 days (with repetitive treatments if necessary)	Improved reoperation rate for endoscopic sinus surgery
Chang et al. [38]	Ivacaftor	10 months	Improved symptoms and FEV1
Lindstrom et al. [40]	Ibuprofen	Unknown	Temporary resolution of nasal polyps with >50% of patients experiencing recurrence

Abbreviations, LKNE: Lund–Kennedy Nasal Endoscopy, LMS: Lund–Mackay score, FEV1: forced expiratory volume in 1 s, SNOT-22: Sinonasal Outcome Test-22.

Ibuprofen is yet another medical therapy that some have trialed for the treatment of CF-related sinonasal disease. One study showed that 12 patients with CF and nasal polyposis had resolution of their nasal polyps at some point during high-dose ibuprofen therapy [42]. However, more than half of patients who stopped ibuprofen had a recurrence of nasal polyps, likely indicating only a temporary benefit [40]. While multiple studies have shown a pulmonary benefit in the use of ibuprofen for CF patients, studies evaluating its use in concordant CRS are limited to this one study that at best indicates a partial temporary response to nasal polyposis [43,44].

Our Experience

At our institution, we use a variety of methods to diagnose and treat patients with CF CRS. Our main diagnostic strategies include history, physical exam, nasal endoscopy, and CT of the paranasal sinuses to evaluate for mucosal inflammation and presence of sinus hypoplasia/and osteitic bone. Together, our otolaryngologists and pulmonologists additionally discuss recent pulmonary function and frequency of pulmonary infections to help determine which patients may require treatment. Our therapeutic strategy includes a combination of surgical and medical therapy; the details of surgical therapy are outside the scope of this review. The medical management includes a combination of saline irrigation compounded with a corticosteroid and antibiotics, delivered with a sinus rinse bottle, which is readily available at local pharmacies. Our experience is consistent with the benefits demonstrated in the literature regarding similar strategies. Additionally, many patients referred to our office are concurrently using systemic therapies such as a *CFTR* modulator.

6. Conclusions

Cystic fibrosis is a multisystem disease with a high-level of pulmonary morbidity and mortality that also has a considerable impact on the paranasal sinuses. CRS negatively affects quality of life in individuals with CF. Defining CF-related sinonasal disease and determining the indications for medical and surgical intervention remain a challenge. For primary medical therapy to treat CF-related sinus disease, a range of options are available, with the most data supporting the use of dornase alfa, topical corticosteroids, and topical antibiotics. Further prospective trials are needed to determine the optimal medical management for these patients.

Funding: This research received no external funding.

Conflicts of Interest: The authors declare no conflict of interest.

References

1. Mainz, J.G.; Koitschev, A. Pathogenesis and management of nasal polyposis in cystic fibrosis. *Curr. Allergy Asthma Rep.* **2012**, *12*, 163–174. [CrossRef] [PubMed]
2. Rey, M.M.; Bonk, M.P.; Hadjiliadis, D. Cystic Fibrosis: Emerging Understanding and Therapies. *Annu. Rev. Med.* **2019**, *70*, 197–210. [CrossRef]
3. Tipirneni, K.E.; Woodworth, B.A. Medical and surgical advancements in the management of cystic fibrosis chronic rhinosinusitis. *Curr. Otorhinolaryngol. Rep.* **2017**, *5*, 24–34. [CrossRef] [PubMed]
4. Illing, E.A.; Woodworth, B.A. Management of the upper airway in cystic fibrosis. *Curr. Opin. Pulm. Med.* **2014**, *20*, 623–631. [CrossRef]
5. Johansen, H.K.; Aanaes, K.; Pressler, T.; Nielsen, K.G.; Fisker, J.; Skov, M.; Høiby, N.; von Buchwald, C. Colonisation and infection of the paranasal sinuses in cystic fibrosis patients is accompanied by a reduced PMN response. *J. Cyst. Fibros.* **2012**, *11*, 525–531. [CrossRef] [PubMed]
6. Alanin, M.C.; Aanaes, K.; Høiby, N.; Pressler, T.; Skov, M.; Nielsen, K.G.; Taylor-Robinson, D.; Waldmann, E.; Krogh, H.J. Sinus surgery postpones chronic Gram-negative lung infection: Cohort study of 106 patients with cystic fibrosis. *Rhinology* **2016**, *54*, 206–213. [CrossRef] [PubMed]
7. Orlandi, R.R.; Kingdom, T.T.; Hwang, P.H.; Smith, T.L.; Alt, J.A.; Baroody, F.M.; Batra, P.S.; Bernal-Sprekelsen, M.; Bhattacharyya, N.; Chandra, R.K.; et al. International consensus statement on allergy and rhinology: Rhinosinusitis. *Int. Forum Allergy Rhinol.* **2016**, *6*, S22–S209. [CrossRef] [PubMed]
8. Berkhout, M.C.; Van Rooden, C.J.; Rijntjes, E.; Fokkens, W.J.; El Bouazzaoui, L.H.; Heijerman, H.G. Sinonasal manifestations of cystic fibrosis: A correlation between genotype and phenotype? *J. Cyst. Fibros.* **2014**, *13*, 442–448. [CrossRef]
9. Hopkins, C.; Gillett, S.; Slack, R.; Lund, V.J.; Browne, J.P. Psychometric validity of the 22-item Sinonasal Outcome Test. *Clin. Otolaryngol.* **2009**, *34*, 447–454. [CrossRef]
10. Habib, A.R.; Quon, B.S.; Buxton, J.A.; Alsaleh, S.; Singer, J.; Manji, J.; Wicox, P.G.; Javer, A.R. The Sino-Nasal Outcome Test–22 as a tool to identify chronic rhinosinusitis in adults with cystic fibrosis. *Int. Forum Allergy Rhinol.* **2015**, *5*, 1111–1117. [CrossRef]
11. Habib, A.R.; Buxton, J.A.; Singer, J.; Wilcox, P.G.; Javer, A.R.; Quon, B.S. Association between chronic rhinosinusitis and health-related quality of life in adults with cystic fibrosis. *Ann. Am. Thorac. Soc.* **2015**, *12*, 1163–1169. [CrossRef] [PubMed]
12. Kay, D.J.; Rosenfeld, R.M. Quality of life for children with persistent sinonasal symptoms. *Otolaryngol. Head Neck Surg.* **2003**, *128*, 17–26. [CrossRef] [PubMed]
13. Wentzel, J.L.; Virella-Lowell, I.; Schlosser, R.J.; Soler, Z.M. Quantitative sinonasal symptom assessment in an unselected pediatric population with cystic fibrosis. *Am. J. Rhinol. Allergy* **2015**, *29*, 357–361. [CrossRef] [PubMed]
14. Xie, D.X.; Wu, J.; Kelly, K.; Brown, R.F.; Shannon, C.; Virgin, F.W. Evaluating the sinus and Nasal Quality of Life Survey in the pediatric cystic fibrosis patient population. *Int. J. Pediatr. Otorhinolaryngol.* **2017**, *102*, 133–137. [CrossRef] [PubMed]
15. Casserly, P.; Harrison, M.; O'Connell, O.; O'Donovan, N.; Plant, B.J.; O'Sullivan, P. Nasal endoscopy and paranasal sinus computerised tomography (CT) findings in an Irish cystic fibrosis adult patient group. *Eur. Arch. Oto-Rhino-Laryngol.* **2015**, *272*, 3353–3359. [CrossRef] [PubMed]
16. Kang, S.H.; Piltcher, O.B.; de Tarso Roth Dalcin, P. Sinonasal alterations in computed tomography scans in cystic fibrosis: A literature review of observational studies. *Int. Forum Allergy Rhinol.* **2014**, *4*, 223–231. [CrossRef] [PubMed]
17. Berkhout, M.C.; Klerx-Melis, F.; Fokkens, W.J.; Nuijsink, M.; van Aalderen, W.M.; Heijerman, H.G. CT-abnormalities, bacteriology and symptoms of sinonasal disease in children with Cystic Fibrosis. *J. Cyst. Fibros.* **2016**, *15*, 816–824. [CrossRef] [PubMed]
18. Orlandi, R.R.; Wiggins, R.H., III. Radiological sinonasal findings in adults with cystic fibrosis. *Am. J. Rhinol. Allergy* **2009**, *23*, 307–311. [CrossRef]
19. Rasmussen, J.; Aanæs, K.; Norling, R.; Nielsen, K.G.; Johansen, H.K.; von Buchwald, C. CT of the paranasal sinuses is not a valid indicator for sinus surgery in CF patients. *J. Cyst. Fibros.* **2012**, *11*, 93–99. [CrossRef]

20. Sheikh, S.I.; Handly, B.; Ryan-Wenger, N.A.; Hayes, D., Jr.; Kirkby, S.E.; McCoy, K.S.; Lind, M. Novel computed tomography scoring system for sinus disease in adults with cystic fibrosis. *Ann. Otol. Rhinol. Laryngol.* **2016**, *125*, 838–843. [CrossRef]
21. Gergin, O.; Kawai, K.; MacDougall, R.D.; Robson, C.D.; Moritz, E.; Cunningham, M.; Adil, E. Sinus Computed Tomography Imaging in Pediatric Cystic Fibrosis: Added Value? *Otolaryngol. Head Neck Surg.* **2016**, *155*, 160–165. [CrossRef] [PubMed]
22. Abuzeid, W.M.; Song, C.; Fastenberg, J.H.; Fang, C.H.; Ayoub, N.; Jerschow, E.; Mohabir, P.K.; Hwang, P.H. Correlations between cystic fibrosis genotype and sinus disease severity in chronic rhinosinusitis. *Laryngoscope* **2018**, *128*, 1752–1758. [CrossRef] [PubMed]
23. Mainz, J.G.; Koitschev, A. Management of chronic rhinosinusitis in CF. *J. Cyst. Fibros.* **2009**, *8*, S10–S14. [CrossRef]
24. Cimmino, M.; Nardone, M.; Cavaliere, M.; Plantulli, A.; Sepe, A.; Esposito, V.; Mazzarella, G.; Raia, V. Dornase alfa as postoperative therapy in cystic fibrosis sinonasal disease. *Arch. Otolaryngol. Head Neck Surg.* **2005**, *131*, 1097–1101. [CrossRef] [PubMed]
25. Mainz, J.G.; Schien, C.; Schiller, I.; Schädlich, K.; Koitschev, A.; Koitschev, C.; Riethmüller, J.; Graepler-Mainka, U.; Wiedemann, B.; Beck, J.F. Sinonasal inhalation of dornase alfa administered by vibrating aerosol to cystic fibrosis patients: A double-blind placebo-controlled cross-over trial. *J. Cyst. Fibros.* **2014**, *13*, 461–470. [CrossRef] [PubMed]
26. Mainz, J.G.; Schumacher, U.; Schädlich, K.; Hentschel, J.; Koitschev, C.; Koitschev, A.; Riethmüller, J.; Prenzel, F.; Sommerburg, O.; Wiedemann, B.; et al. Sino nasal inhalation of isotonic versus hypertonic saline (6.0%) in CF patients with chronic rhinosinusitis—Results of a multicenter, prospective, randomized, double-blind, controlled trial. *J. Cyst. Fibros.* **2016**, *15*, e57–e66. [CrossRef] [PubMed]
27. Aanaes, K.; Alanin, M.C.; Nielsen, K.G.; Møller, M.J.; Høiby, N.; Johansen, H.K.; Johannesen, H.H.; Mortensen, J. The accessibility of topical treatment in the paranasal sinuses on operated cystic fibrosis patients assessed by scintigraphy. *Rhinology* **2018**, *56*, 268–273. [CrossRef]
28. Hadfield, P.J.; Rowe-Jones, J.M.; Mackay, I.S. A prospective treatment trial of nasal polyps in adults with cystic fibrosis. *Rhinology* **2000**, *38*, 63–65.
29. Donaldson, J.D.; Gillespie, C.T. Observations on the efficacy of intranasal beclomethasone dipropionate in cystic fibrosis patients. *J. Otolaryngol.* **1988**, *17*, 43–45.
30. Costantini, D.; Di, M.C.; Giunta, A.; Amabile, G. Nasal polyposis in cystic fibrosis treated by beclomethasone dipropionate. *Acta Univ. Carol. Med.* **1990**, *36*, 220–221.
31. Pignataro, L.D.; Di Cicco, M.; Gaini, R.M.; Amabile, G.; Costantini, D. Beclomethasone dipropionate in the treatment of nasal polyps of cystic fibrosis patients: Four years follow-up. *Riv. Ital. Otorinolaringol. Audiol. Foniatr.* **1993**, *13*, 65–66.
32. Welch, K.C.; Thaler, E.R.; Doghramji, L.L.; Palmer, J.N.; Chiu, A.G. The effects of serum and urinary cortisol levels of topical intranasal irrigations with budesonide added to saline in patients with recurrent polyposis after endoscopic sinus surgery. *Am. J. Rhinol. Allergy* **2010**, *24*, 26–28. [CrossRef] [PubMed]
33. Bhalla, R.K.; Payton, K.; Wright, E.D. Safety of budesonide in saline sinonasal irrigations in the management of chronic rhinosinusitis with polyposis: Lack of significant adrenal suppression. *J. Otolaryngol. Head Neck Surg.* **2008**, *37*, 821. [PubMed]
34. Mainz, J.G.; Naehrlich, L.; Schien, M.; Käding, M.; Schiller, I.; Mayr, S.; Schneider, G.; Wiehlmann, L.; Cramer, N.; Pfister, W.; et al. Concordant genotype of upper and lower airways *P. aeruginosa* and *S. aureus* isolates in cystic fibrosis. *Thorax* **2009**, *64*, 535–540. [CrossRef] [PubMed]
35. Aanaes, K.; von Buchwald, C.; Hjuler, T.; Skov, M.; Alanin, M.; Johansen, H.K. The effect of sinus surgery with intensive follow-up on pathogenic sinus bacteria in patients with cystic fibrosis. *Am. J. Rhinol. Allergy* **2013**, *27*, e1–e4. [CrossRef] [PubMed]
36. Mainz, J.G.; Schädlich, K.; Schien, C.; Michl, R.; Schelhorn-Neise, P.; Koitschev, A.; Koitschev, C.; Keller, P.M.; Riethmüller, J.; Wiedemann, B.; et al. Sinonasal inhalation of tobramycin vibrating aerosol in cystic fibrosis patients with upper airway *Pseudomonas aeruginosa* colonization: Results of a randomized, double-blind, placebo-controlled pilot study. *Drug Des. Dev. Ther.* **2014**, *8*, 209. [CrossRef] [PubMed]
37. Moss, R.B.; King, V.V. Management of sinusitis in cystic fibrosis by endoscopic surgery and serial antimicrobial lavage: Reduction in recurrence requiring surgery. *Arch. Otolaryngol. Head Neck Surg.* **1995**, *121*, 566–572. [CrossRef] [PubMed]

38. Chang, E.H.; Tang, X.X.; Shah, V.S.; Launspach, J.L.; Ernst, S.E.; Hilkin, B.; Karp, P.H.; Abou Alaiwa, M.H.; Graham, S.M.; Hornick, D.B.; et al. Medical reversal of chronic sinusitis in a cystic fibrosis patient with ivacaftor. *Int. Forum Allergy Rhinol.* **2015**, *5*, 178–181. [CrossRef]
39. Sawicki, G.S.; McKone, E.F.; Pasta, D.J.; Millar, S.J.; Wagener, J.S.; Johnson, C.A.; Konstan, M.W. Sustained benefit from ivacaftor demonstrated by combining clinical trial and cystic fibrosis patient registry data. *Am. J. Respir. Crit. Care Med.* **2015**, *192*, 836–842. [CrossRef]
40. Ramsey, B.W.; Davies, J.; McElvaney, N.G.; Tullis, E.; Bell, S.C.; Dřevínek, P.; Griese, M.; McKone, E.F.; Wainwright, C.E.; Konstan, M.W.; et al. A CFTR potentiator in patients with cystic fibrosis and the G551D mutation. *N. Engl. J. Med.* **2011**, *365*, 1663–1672. [CrossRef]
41. McCormick, J.; Cho, D.Y.; Lampkin, B.; Richman, J.; Hathorne, H.; Rowe, S.M.; Woodworth, B.A. Ivacaftor improves rhinologic, psychologic, and sleep-related quality of life in G551D cystic fibrosis patients. *Int. Forum Allergy Rhinol.* **2018**. [CrossRef] [PubMed]
42. Lindstrom, D.R.; Conley, S.F.; Splaingard, M.L.; Gershan, W.M. Ibuprofen therapy and nasal polyposis in cystic fibrosis patients. *J. Otolaryngol.* **2007**, *36*, 309–314. [CrossRef] [PubMed]
43. Konstan, M.W.; VanDevanter, D.R.; Sawicki, G.S.; Pasta, D.J.; Foreman, A.J.; Neiman, E.A.; Morgan, W.J. Association of high-dose ibuprofen use, lung function decline, and long-term survival in children with cystic fibrosis. *Ann. Am. Thorac. Soc.* **2018**, *15*, 485–493. [CrossRef] [PubMed]
44. Lands, L.C.; Stanojevic, S. Oral non-steroidal anti-inflammatory drug therapy for lung disease in cystic fibrosis. *Cochrane Database Syst. Rev.* **2016**, *4*, CD001505. [CrossRef] [PubMed]

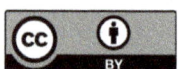

© 2019 by the authors. Licensee MDPI, Basel, Switzerland. This article is an open access article distributed under the terms and conditions of the Creative Commons Attribution (CC BY) license (http://creativecommons.org/licenses/by/4.0/).

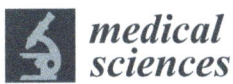

Review

Chronic Rhinosinusitis: Does Allergy Play a Role?

Sonya Marcus, John M. DelGaudio, Lauren T. Roland and Sarah K. Wise *

Department of Otolaryngology-Head and Neck Surgery, Emory University, Atlanta, GA 30308, USA; sonya.marcus@emory.edu (S.M.); jdelgau@emory.edu (J.M.D.); lauren.roland@emory.edu (L.T.R.)
* Correspondence: skmille@emory.edu; Tel.: +1-404-686-1424

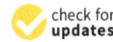

Received: 13 January 2019; Accepted: 12 February 2019; Published: 18 February 2019

Abstract: A few chronic rhinosinusitis (CRS) variants have demonstrated a strong association with environmental allergy, including allergic fungal rhinosinusitis (AFRS) and central compartment atopic disease (CCAD). However, the overall relationship between CRS and allergy remains poorly defined. The goal of this review is to evaluate the relationship between CRS and allergy with a focus on specific CRS variants.

Keywords: allergy; chronic rhinosinusitis; polyposis; allergic fungal rhinosinusitis; central compartment atopic disease

1. Introduction

Chronic rhinosinusitis (CRS) is an inflammatory condition within the paranasal sinuses that persists for more than 12 weeks [1]. It affects approximately 5% of the US population, with an estimated overall direct cost burden of about US $8.6 billion per year [2]. Given this substantial societal burden, significant research has been dedicated to better understanding CRS.

In recent decades, we have gained an increased understanding that CRS is not a uniform disease process but rather encompasses several different phenotypes and endotypes [3]. Historically, CRS has been divided into two main phenotypes: CRS with nasal polyposis (CRSwNP) and CRS without nasal polyposis (CRSsNP). However, within these broad phenotypes, various endotypes exist. For example, within the CRSwNP patient population, allergic fungal rhinosinusitis (AFRS) and aspirin exacerbated respiratory disease (AERD) represent clinically distinct entities requiring differing management.

Furthermore, CRS is a multifactorial disease process with genetic, environmental, bacterial and immunologic contributions, among other etiologies. In addition, allergic diseases, especially immunoglobulin E (IgE)-mediated inflammatory processes such as allergic rhinitis (AR) may influence the development and progression of CRS and should be considered in the CRS work-up and management [4]. However, the role of allergy as a comorbidity for CRS remains incompletely understood and appears to have a greater association with certain CRS endotypes.

Therefore, the goal of this review is to examine the relationship between allergy and CRS, with a focus on specific CRS endotypes.

2. Association between Allergic Rhinitis and Chronic Rhinosinusitis: Overview

There are several proposed mechanisms by which allergy may contribute to CRS. Yet, despite evidence regarding a pathophysiologic association, clinical studies demonstrating a relationship between allergy and CRS have been conflicting [5], especially when patients are subtyped by broad phenotypic categories (CRSwNP and CRSsNP).

There is, however, strong evidence for an association with certain CRS subtypes, including allergic fungal rhinosinusitis (AFRS) and the more recently described central compartment atopic disease (CCAD), which will be individually discussed within this review.

3. Association between Allergic Rhinitis and Chronic Rhinosinusitis: Pathophysiology

Significant study has been dedicated toward better understanding the inflammatory profiles that contribute to the development and propagation of CRS. Broadly, CRS has been divided into CRSwNP and CRSsNP, but further classification is based upon association with a type 1 or type 2 inflammatory pattern. Type 1 inflammation is characterized by the presence of neutrophils and type 1 cytokines, such as interferon-γ (IFN-γ). Type 2 inflammation is characterized by the presence of eosinophils and type 2 cytokines, such as interleukin 4 (IL-4), IL-5 and IL-13. Traditionally, CRSsNP has been associated with type 1 inflammation and CRSwNP with type 2 inflammation. However, eosinophilia has also been shown to be present in CRSsNP [6]. In addition, the traditional type 1 vs. type 2 delineation does not tell the whole story. The roles of IL-17, IL-21, IL-22, IL-26, innate lymphoid cells, and other cellular and soluble mediators are being increasingly recognized in CRS pathophysiology [7–9].

Allergy is also characterized by type 2 inflammation and because of this similarity, an association between allergy and CRS (more specifically CRSwNP) has frequently been assumed. However, the mechanisms by which allergy may influence CRS are not inherently obvious. Although allergens enter the nose via inspiration, inspiration alone cannot introduce allergens into the sinuses. A study by Adkins et al. [10] using radiolabeled ragweed pollen and subsequent imaging demonstrated that allergen particles were unable to enter the paranasal sinuses despite being present within the nasal cavity and oropharynx. Furthermore, inflammation and polyposis cause meatal obstruction, which would make direct entry of aeroallergens into the sinuses difficult.

When allergy plays a significant role in CRS, some evidence points to a systemic process as a potential mechanism. In a sensitized patient, aeroallergens engage nasal dendritic cells, which then activate effector T-helper lymphocytes. Aeroallergens can also be processed by non-professional antigen-presenting cells such as macrophages, B-lymphocytes, mast cells and eosinophils within the nasal cavities to activate allergen-specific effector T lymphocytes [11]. These cells then migrate to the bone marrow. Once in the bone marrow, cytokines associated with allergic inflammation, including IL-4, IL-5 and IL-13, are released which stimulate the production of eosinophils, mast cells and basophils which enter the systemic circulation and recognize adhesion molecules and chemotactic signals. It is via this mechanism that eosinophilia progresses within the nasal cavities following seasonal aeroallergen exposure [12]. However, eosinophils will also be directed into tissues that display relevant adhesion molecules and chemotactic signals. Chronic rhinosinusitis patients express the necessary adhesion molecules and chemotactic machinery to recruit inflammatory cells into the sinuses [13,14], and it is by this mechanism that allergens may exacerbate CRS. A study by Baroody et al. [15] substantiated the concept of a systemic process linking allergy with CRS. Upon performing unilateral nasal allergen challenge, eosinophilia was increased not only in the ipsilateral maxillary sinus but in the contralateral maxillary sinus as well.

In a subset of patients, however, systemic allergy testing is negative but locally-present IgE in the sinonasal cavity may be present, a condition that has been referred to as local allergic rhinitis (LAR) or entopy. The immunological characteristics of LAR are local IgE production, type 2 inflammation and a positive nasal provocation allergen test. Immunoglobin class switching to IgE has been demonstrated in the nasal mucosa, so there is also a plausible mechanism for allergic processes completely confined to the nasal tissues, without systemic involvement [16–18].

Overall, these findings demonstrate a potential pathophysiologic link between aeroallergen exposure and CRS. However, further study is necessary to understand the relationship between local and systemic allergic inflammation. Also of note, the majority of the aforementioned studies pertain to patients with eosinophilic chronic rhinosinusitis (with nasal polyposis). The systemic and local mechanisms contributing to other phenotypes, including AFRS and CCAD, need further elucidation.

4. Evidence for a Link between Allergic Rhinitis and Chronic Rhinosinusitis: Clinical Evidence

Despite some evidence of pathophysiologic overlap between allergy and CRS, clinical studies have demonstrated contradictory findings. Wilson et al. [5] performed the most comprehensive systematic review evaluating the relationship between allergy and CRS. Twenty-four articles were included in this review. Nearly an equal number of studies supported or refuted an association of allergy with CRS in patients with CRSwNP or CRSsNP.

4.1. Chronic Rhinosinusitis with Nasal Polyposis

CRSwNP is strongly associated with Th2-mediated inflammation [19], as is allergy. In fact, several studies have supported a relationship by demonstrating increased rates of positive skin prick testing (SPT) among CRSwNP patients compared to controls [20,21]. However, several other studies have demonstrated no significant relationship. For example, Erbeck et al. [22] demonstrated no relationship between allergy and polyp size, symptoms or recurrence rate. In the aforementioned review article by Wilson et al. [3], ten studies supported an association between CRSwNP and allergy while seven did not. One study was equivocal. Therefore, despite some overlapping pathophysiologic features, conflicting data exists regarding a relationship between allergy and CRSwNP.

4.2. Chronic Rhinosinusitis without Nasal Polyposis

Fewer studies have evaluated the relationship between CRSsNP and allergy. Some studies have suggested a higher burden of sinonasal disease in allergic patients based on imaging [23,24]. However, other studies have demonstrated no association [25]. In the article by Wilson et al. [3], four studies supported an association between allergy and CRSsNP and five did not. Again, this demonstrates conflicting data regarding a relationship between allergy and CRSsNP.

Given these findings, Wilson et al. and subsequently The International Consensus Statement on Allergy and Rhinology: Allergic Rhinitis concluded that the aggregate level of evidence linking allergy to either CRS subtype was level D [4,5]. However, significant limitations exist within the prior literature. First, studies often included patients with and without polyposis in the same cohort [26,27]. Second, even amongst patients with polyposis, certain CRS endotypes may be more closely associated with allergen exposure than others. Yet, it was often not clarified whether these endotypes were included within or excluded from the study cohort, thus potentially skewing the analysis in one direction or the other. For instance, two CRS subtypes that have shown a greater association with allergy are AFRS and the more recently described CCAD, which will both be individually discussed.

5. Subtypes of CRS Demonstrating a Link between Allergic Rhinitis and Chronic Rhinosinusitis

5.1. Allergic Fungal Rhinosinusitis

Allergic fungal rhinosinusitis (AFRS) is a noninvasive, recurrent subset of CRSwNP that most commonly affects immunocompetent hosts. It is most prevalent within the Mississippi river basin, and southern regions of the United States [28]. In 1994, Bent and Kuhn published five major criteria to establish the diagnosis of AFRS, one of which is a type I hypersensitivity to inhaled fungal elements confirmed by history, skin testing or serology. Therefore by definition, patients with AFRS have allergy. Since then, the role of allergy in AFRS has been reinforced, and sometimes questioned, within the literature. Manning and Holman [29] compared culture-positive *Bipolaris* AFRS patients to non-CRS patients and found *Bipolaris*-specific IgE and IgG antibodies, as well as positive skin prick testing to *Bipolaris* in patients with AFRS. Furthermore, the largest AFRS case series reported from the southwestern United States found that all patients with AFRS had inhalant allergy [30]. However, not all patients with fungal allergy develop AFRS, and conversely not all patients with AFRS demonstrate fungal allergy, raising questions regarding the pathogenesis of this entity [31]. One possible theory to explain the absence of fungal allergy was suggested by Collins et al., who proposed that AFRS might result from a local, rather than a systemic, allergic process [32].

5.2. Central Compartment Atopic Disease (CCAD)

Central compartment atopic disease (CCAD) is a more recently described CRS variant strongly associated with allergy. First described in 2014 [33], although not yet named CCAD, this variant includes polypoid changes of the middle turbinate. In this study, all twenty-five patients tested positive for inhalant allergy. Brunner et al. [34] similarly demonstrated a higher association of allergen sensitization in patients with isolated middle turbinate changes than in those with diffuse polyposis. Later, additional clinical description of this entity, including more advanced forms, was published [35], demonstrating that other central structures including the posterior–superior nasal septum, middle turbinates, and superior turbinates are involved. In this study, 14/15 patients tested positive for inhalant allergies. Hamizan et al. [36] evaluated radiologic findings associated with CCAD, and found that a central pattern of mucosal disease had a higher association with allergy. Overall, this central pattern of inflammatory changes has been shown to have a high association with allergy. Further study is needed to better clarify the etiology and clinical course of this CRS subtype.

6. Management

If allergy contributes to CRS, then it would be logical that allergen-targeting therapies would be efficacious in the treatment of CRS. Such treatments include immunotherapy, anti-IgE, and anti-cytokine (IL-4, IL-5, IL-13) therapy, which will be discussed.

6.1. Immunotherapy

Despite a strong recommendation for allergen immunotherapy (IT) in patients with allergic rhinitis (AR), its role in CRS remains less certain. A systematic review by DeYoung et al. [37] looked at sinusitis-specific outcomes in CRS patients who underwent IT. Seven studies were included which demonstrated symptom reduction in the short-term, however the number and quality of studies included deemed this conclusion to be weak. Current CRS treatment recommendations specify allergy testing and treatment as an option.

The role of IT in the treatment of AFRS has also been examined. For instance, Folker et al. [38] demonstrated decreased severity of patient symptoms after receiving IT. Yet overall, studies that have examined the role of allergen-specific immunotherapy in the treatment of AFRS have a relatively low level of evidence. Furthermore, a more recent evidence-based review by Gan et al. [39] concluded, based on a limited number of studies, that there was an equal degree of benefit and harm, and that IT should only be considered as an option for AFRS. The role of immunotherapy in CCAD has not yet been studied.

6.2. Anti-Immunoglobulin E Therapy

Omalizumab is an IgE-targeting therapy, which selectively binds free circulating IgE and decreases the expression of IgE receptors on mast cells, basophils, and dendritic cells. Prior studies have demonstrated its efficacy in the management of recalcitrant CRSwNP [40]. Symptom improvement after treatment with IgE-targeting therapies would provide a compelling argument for the role of allergy in CRS. However, evidence for its efficacy remains mixed and the mechanism of action by which omalizumab is effective in patients with CRSwNP is still being elucidated. Gevaert et al. [41] found significant reduction of polyp size and quality of life improvement with anti-IgE therapy. However, they showed that this improvement was related to local mucosal IgE levels and not total serum IgE level. Therefore, the authors felt that its efficacy may be related to increased local tissue IgE, associated with Staphylococcus aureus enterotoxin, rather than inhalant allergy. Pinto et al. [42] showed non-statistically significant improvements on imaging and Sino-Nasal Outcome Test (SNOT-20) measures after treatment with omalizumab and concluded that IgE only played a small role in the mucosal inflammation of CRS. Therefore, the evidence remains mixed.

6.3. Anti-Cytokine Therapy

Allergy is characterized by a type 2 inflammatory pattern, which includes cytokines IL-4, IL-5 and IL-13. Symptom improvement after treatment with therapies directed at these cytokines would provide additional evidence for the contribution of allergy to CRS. A recent systematic review by Tsetsos et al. [43] evaluated the efficacy of such therapies in patients with CRSwNP. This review included randomized controlled trials, which evaluated anti-IL-5 (reslizumab and mepolizumab) and anti-IL-4/IL-13 (dupilumbab) biologics. Overall, results were encouraging despite the inclusion of few studies with small sample sizes. Reslizumab was shown to reduce nasal polyp size, but only in patients with elevated nasal IL-5 levels [44]. Mepolizumab was found to reduce the need for surgery in CRSwNP patients [45], and dupilumab was found to reduce nasal polyp burden [46].

7. Conclusions

Despite an assumed association between allergy and CRS, evidence for a relationship remains debated, especially when patients are subtyped into the broad classification of CRSwNP and CRSsNP. Certain CRS endotypes, however, have demonstrated a stronger association with allergy, including allergic fungal rhinosinusitis (AFRS) and central compartment atopic disease (CCAD). Thus, it is likely that with better-defined CRS categorization, we will be able to better delineate the relationship between allergy and specific CRS endotypes in the future.

Author Contributions: Writing—Original Draft Preparation, S.M. and S.K.W. Review and Editing, S.M., L.T.R., J.M.D. and S.K.W. Review and Approval of Final Draft, S.M., L.T.R., J.M.D. and S.K.W.

Funding: This research received no external funding.

Conflicts of Interest: The authors declare no conflict of interest.

References

1. Benninger, M.S.; Ferguson, B.J.; Hadley, J.A.; Hamilos, D.L.; Jacobs, M.; Kennedy, D.W.; Lanza, D.C.; Marple, B.F.; Osguthorpe, J.D.; Stankiewicz, J.A.; et al. Adult chronic rhinosinusitis: Definitions, diagnosis, epidemiology, and pathophysiology. *Otolaryngol. Head Neck Surg.* **2003**, *129* (Suppl. 3), S1–S32. [CrossRef] [PubMed]
2. Bhattacharyya, N. Incremental health care utilization and expenditures for chronic rhinosinusitis in the United States. *Ann. Otol. Rhinol. Laryngol.* **2011**, *120*, 423–427. [CrossRef] [PubMed]
3. Gurrola, J., 2nd.; Borish, L. Chronic Rhinosinusitis: Endotypes, biomarkers, and treatment response. *J. Allergy Clin. Immunol.* **2017**, *140*, 1499–1508. [CrossRef]
4. Wise, S.K.; Lin, S.Y.; Toskala, E.; Orlandi, R.R.; Akdis, C.A.; Alt, J.A.; Azar, A.; Baroody, F.M.; Bachert, C.; Canonica, G.W. International Consensus Statement on Allergy and Rhinology: Allergic Rhinitis. *Int. Forum Allergy Rhinol.* **2018**, *8*, 108–352. [CrossRef] [PubMed]
5. Wilson, K.F.; McMains, C.; Orlandi, R.F. The association between allergy and chronic rhinosinusitis with and without nasal polyposis: An evidence-based review with recommendations. *Int. Forum Allergy Rhinol.* **2014**, *4*, 93–103. [CrossRef] [PubMed]
6. Lam, K.; Kern, R.C.; Luong, A. Is there a future for biologics in the management of chronic rhinosinusitis? *Int. Forum Allergy Rhinol.* **2016**, *6*, 935–942. [CrossRef] [PubMed]
7. Miljkovic, D.; Psaltis, A.J.; Wormald, P.J.; Vreugde, S. Chronic rhinosinusitis with polyps is characterized by increased mucosal and blood Th17 effector cytokine producing cells. *Front. Physiol.* **2017**, *19*, 898. [CrossRef] [PubMed]
8. Ramezanpour, M.; Moraitis, S.; Smith, J.L.; Wormald, P.J.; Vreugde, S. Th17 Cytokines Disrupt the Airway Mucosal Barrier in Chronic Rhinosinusitis. *Med. Inflamm.* **2016**, *2016*, 1–7. [CrossRef] [PubMed]
9. Kato, A. Immunopathology of chronic rhinosinusitis. *Allergol. Int.* **2015**, *64*, 121–130. [CrossRef]
10. Adkins, T.N.; Goodgold, H.M.; Hendershott, L.; Slavin, R.G. Does inhaled pollen enter the sinus cavities? *Ann. Allergy Asthma Immunol.* **1998**, *81*, 181–184. [CrossRef]
11. Kennedy, J.L.; Borish, L. Chronic sinusitis pathophysiology: The role of allergy. *Am. J. Rhinol.* **2013**, *27*, 367–371. [CrossRef] [PubMed]

12. Minshall, E.M.; Cameron, L.; Lavigne, F.; Leung, D.Y.; Hamilos, D.; Garcia-Zepada, E.A.; Rothenberg, M.; Luster, A.D.; Hamid, Q. Eotaxin mRNA and protein expression in chronic sinusitis and allergen-induced nasal responses in seasonal allergic rhinitis. *Am. J. Respir. Cell Mol. Biol.* **1997**, *17*, 683–690. [CrossRef] [PubMed]
13. Jahnsen, F.L.; Haraldsen, G.; Aanesen, J.P.; Haye, R.; Brandtzaeg, P. Eosinophil infiltration is related to increased expression of vascular cell adhesion molecule-1 in nasal polyps. *Am. J. Respir. Cell Mol. Biol.* **1995**, *12*, 624–632. [CrossRef] [PubMed]
14. Inman, M.D.; Ellis, R.; Wattie, J.; Denburg, J.A.; O'Byrne, P.M. Allergen-induced increase in airway responsiveness, airway eosinophilia, and bone-marrow eosinophil progenitors in mice. *Am. J. Respir. Cell Mol. Biol.* **1999**, *21*, 473–479. [CrossRef] [PubMed]
15. Baroody, F.M.; Mucha, S.M.; Detineo, M.; Neclerio, R.M. Nasal challenge with allergen leads to maxillary sinus inflammation. *J. Allergy Clin. Immunol.* **2008**, *121*, 1126–1132. [CrossRef] [PubMed]
16. Smurthwaite, L.; Durham, S.R. Local IgE synthesis in allergic rhinitis and asthma. *Curr. Allergy Asthma Rep.* **2002**, *2*, 231–238. [CrossRef] [PubMed]
17. Wise, S.K.; Ahn, C.N.; Schlosser, R.J. Localized immunoglobulin E expression in allergic rhinitis and nasal polyposis. *Curr. Opin. Otolaryngol. Head Neck Surg.* **2009**, *17*, 216–222. [CrossRef]
18. Gevaert, P.; Holtappels, G.; Johansson, S.G.; Cuvelier, C.; Cauwenberge, P.; Bachert, C. Organization of secondary lymphoid tissue and local IgE formation to Staphylococcus aureus enterotoxins in nasal polyp tissue. *Allergy* **2005**, *60*, 71–79. [CrossRef]
19. Orlandi, R.R.; Kingdom, T.T.; Hwang, P.H.; Smith, T.L.; Alt, J.A.; Baroody, F.M.; Batra, P.S.; Bernal-Sprekelsen, M.; Bhattacharyya, N.; Chandra, R.K. International Consensus Statement on Allergy and Rhinology: Rhinosinusitis. *Int. Forum Allergy Rhinol.* **2016**, *6*, S22–S209. [CrossRef]
20. Munoz del Castillo, F.; Jurado-Ramos, A.; Fernandez-Conde, B.L.; Soler, R.; Barasona, M.J.; Cantillo, E.; Moreno, C.; Guerra, F. Allergenic profile of nasal polyposis. *J. Investig. Allergol. Clin. Immunol.* **2009**, *19*, 110–116.
21. Pumhirun, P.; Limitlaohapanth, C.; Wasuwat, P. Role of allergy in nasal polyps of Thai patients. *Asian Pac. J. Allergy Immunol.* **1999**, *17*, 13–15. [PubMed]
22. Erbek, S.; Topal, O.; Cakmak, O. The role of allergy in the severity of nasal polyposis. *Am. J. Rhinol.* **2007**, *21*, 686–690. [CrossRef] [PubMed]
23. Kirtsreesakul, V.; Ruttanaphol, S. The relationship between allergy and rhinosinusitis. *Rhinology* **2008**, *46*, 204–208. [PubMed]
24. Berrettini, S.; Carabelli, A.; Sellari-Franceschini, S.; Bruschini, L.; Abruzzese, A.; Quartieri, F.; Sconosciuto, F. Perennial allergic rhinitis and chronic sinusitis: Correlation with rhinologic risk factors. *Allergy* **1999**, *54*, 242–248. [CrossRef] [PubMed]
25. Gelincik, A.; Buyukozturk, S.; Aslan, I.; Aydin, S.; Ozseker, F.; Colakoglu, B.; Dal, M. Allergic vs. nonallergic rhinitis: Which is more predisposing to chronic rhinosinusitis? *Ann. Allergy Asthma Immunol.* **2008**, *101*, 18–22. [CrossRef]
26. Emanuel, I.A.; Shah, S.B. Chronic rhinosinusitis: Allergy and sinus computed tomography relationships. *Otolaryngol. Head Neck Surg.* **2000**, *123*, 687–691. [CrossRef] [PubMed]
27. Gutman, M.; Torres, A.; Keen, K.J.; Houser, S.M. Prevalence of allergy in patients with chronic rhinosinusitis. *Otolaryngol. Head Neck Surg.* **2004**, *130*, 545–552. [CrossRef] [PubMed]
28. Marple, B.F. Allergic fungal rhinosinusitis: Current theories and management strategies. *Laryngoscope* **2001**, *111*, 1006–1019. [CrossRef] [PubMed]
29. Manning, S.C.; Holman, M. Further evidence for allergic pathophysiology in allergic fungal sinusitis. *Laryngoscope* **1998**, *108*, 1485–1496. [CrossRef] [PubMed]
30. Schubert, M.S.; Goetz, D.W. Evaluation and treatment of allergic fungal sinusitis. I. Demographics and diagnosis. *J. Allergy Clin. Immunol.* **1998**, *102*, 387–394. [CrossRef]
31. Pant, H.; Schembri, M.A.; Wormald, P.J.; Macardle, P.J. IgE-mediated fungal allergy in allergic fungal sinusitis. *Laryngoscope* **2009**, *119*, 1046–1052. [CrossRef] [PubMed]
32. Collins, M.; Nair, S.; Smith, W.; Kette, F.; Gillis, D.; Wormald, P.J. Role of local immunoglobulin E production in the pathophysiology of noninvasive fungal sinusitis. *Laryngoscope* **2004**, *114*, 1242–1246. [CrossRef] [PubMed]

33. White, L.J.; Rotella, M.R.; Delgaudio, J.M. Polypoid changes of the middle turbinate as an indicator of atopic disease. *Int. Forum Allergy Rhinol.* **2014**, *4*, 376–380. [CrossRef] [PubMed]
34. Brunner, J.P.; Jawad, B.A.; McCoul, E.D. Polypoid change of the middle turbinate and paranasal sinus polyposis are distinct entities. *Otolaryngol. Head Neck Surg.* **2017**, *157*, 519–523. [CrossRef] [PubMed]
35. DelGaudio, J.M.; Loftus, P.A.; Hamizan, A.W.; Harvey, R.J.; Wise, S.K. Central compartment atopic disease. *Am. J. Rhinol. Allergy* **2017**, *31*, 228–234. [CrossRef] [PubMed]
36. Hamizan, A.W.; Loftus, P.A.; Alvarado, R.; Ho, J.; Kalish, L.; Sacks, R.; DelGaudio, J.M.; Harvey, R.J. Allergic phenotype of chronic rhinosinusitis based on radiologic pattern of disease. *Laryngoscope* **2018**, *128*, 2015–2021. [CrossRef] [PubMed]
37. De Young, K.; Wentzel, J.L.; Schlosser, R.J.; Nguyen, S.A.; Soler, Z.M. Systematic review of immunotherapy for chronic rhinosinusitis. *Am. J. Rhinol. Allergy* **2014**, *28*, 145–150. [CrossRef] [PubMed]
38. Folker, R.J.; Marple, B.F.; Mabry, R.L.; Mabry, C.S. Treatment of allergic fungal sinusitis: A comparison trial of postoperative immunotherapy with specific fungal antigens. *Laryngoscope* **1998**, *108*, 1623–1627. [CrossRef] [PubMed]
39. Gan, E.C.; Thamboo, A.; Rudmik, L.; Hwang, P.H.; Ferguson, B.J.; Javer, A.R. Medical management of allergic fungal rhinosinusitis following endoscopic sinus surgery: An evidence-based review and recommendations. *Int. Forum Allergy Rhinol.* **2014**, *4*, 702–715. [CrossRef] [PubMed]
40. Bidder, T.; Sahota, J.; Rennie, C.; Lund, V.J.; Robinson, D.S.; Kariyawasam, H.H. Omalizumab treats chronic rhinosinusitis with nasal polyps and asthma together-a real life study. *Rhinology* **2018**, *56*, 42–45. [CrossRef] [PubMed]
41. Gevaert, P.; Calus, L.; Van Zele, T.; Blomme, K.; De Ruyck, N.; Bauters, W.; Hellings, P.; Brusselle, G.; De Bacquer, D.; van Cauwenberge, P. Omalizumab is effective in allergic and nonallergic patients with nasal polyposis and asthma. *J. Allergy Clin. Immunol.* **2013**, *131*, 110–116. [CrossRef] [PubMed]
42. Pinto, J.M.; Mehta, N.A.; di Tineo, M.; Wang, J.; Baroody, F.M.; Naclerio, R.M. A randomized, double-blind, placebo-controlled trial of anti-IgE for chronic rhinosinusitis. *Rhinology* **2010**, *48*, 318–324. [CrossRef] [PubMed]
43. Tsetsos, N.; Goudakos, J.K.; Daskalakis, D.; Konstantinidis, I.; Markou, K. Monoclonal antibodies for the treatment of chronic rhinosinusitis with nasal polyposis. A systematic review. *Rhinology* **2018**, *56*, 11–21. [CrossRef] [PubMed]
44. Gevaert, P.; Lang-Loidolt, D.; Lackner, A.; Stammberger, H.; Staudinger, H.; van Zele, T.; Holtappels, G.; Tavernier, J.; van Cauwenberge, P.; Bachert, C. Nasal IL-5 levels determine the response to anti-IL-5 treatment in patients with nasal polyps. *J. Allergy Clin. Immunol.* **2006**, *118*, 1133–1141. [CrossRef] [PubMed]
45. Bachert, C.; Sousa, A.R.; Lund, V.J.; Scadding, G.K.; Gevaert, P.; Nasser, S.; Durham, S.R.; Cornet, M.E.; Kariyawasam, H.H.; Gilbert, J. Reduced need for surgery in severe nasal polyposis with mepolizumab: Randomized trial. *J. Allergy Clin. Immunol.* **2017**, *140*, 1024–1031. [CrossRef] [PubMed]
46. Bachert, C.; Mannent, L.; Naclerio, R.M.; Mullol, J.; Ferguson, B.J.; Gevaert, P.; Hellings, P.; Jiao, L.; Wang, L.; Evans, R.R. Effect of Subcutaneous Dupilumab on nasal polyp burden in patients with chronic sinusitis and nasal polyposis: A Randomized Clinical Trial. *JAMA* **2016**, *315*, 469–479. [CrossRef] [PubMed]

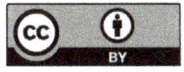

© 2019 by the authors. Licensee MDPI, Basel, Switzerland. This article is an open access article distributed under the terms and conditions of the Creative Commons Attribution (CC BY) license (http://creativecommons.org/licenses/by/4.0/).

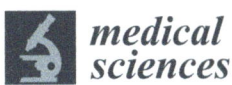

Article

Eosinophilic Upper Airway Inflammation in a Murine Model Using an Adoptive Transfer System Induces Hyposmia and Epithelial Layer Injury with Convex Lesions

Akira Kanda [1,2,*,†], Kenji Kondo [3,†], Naoki Hosaka [4], Yoshiki Kobayashi [1,2], Dan Van Bui [1], Yasutaka Yun [1], Kensuke Suzuki [1], Shunsuke Sawada [1], Mikiya Asako [1,2], Akihiko Nakamura [5], Koichi Tomoda [1], Yoshiko Sakata [6], Koji Tsuta [7], David Dombrowicz [8], Hideyuki Kawauchi [9], Shigeharu Fujieda [10] and Hiroshi Iwai [1]

1. Department of Otolaryngology, Head and Neck Surgery, Kansai Medical University, Hirakata 573-1010, Japan; kobayosh@hirakata.kmu.ac.jp (Y.K.); buivanda@hirakata.kmu.ac.jp (D.V.B.); yunys@hirakata.kmu.ac.jp (Y.Y.); suzukken@hirakata.kmu.ac.jp (K.S.); sawadash@hirakata.kmu.ac.jp (S.S.); asako@hirakata.kmu.ac.jp (M.A.); tomodak@hirakata.kmu.ac.jp (K.T.); iwai@hirakata.kmu.ac.jp (H.I.)
2. Allergy Center, Kansai Medical University, Hirakata 573-1010, Japan
3. Department of Otolaryngology and Head and Neck Surgery, Graduate School of Medicine, the University of Tokyo Hospital, Tokyo, 113-8655, Japan; kondok-tky@umin.ac.jp
4. Department of Pathology, Fuchu Hospital, Izumi 594-0076, Japan; hosakan@hirakata.kmu.ac.jp
5. Nakamura ENT Clinic, Sakai 591-8025, Japan; nakamura-ent@paw.hi-ho.ne.jp
6. Central Research Laboratory, Kansai Medical University, Hirakata 573-1010, Japan; sakatayo@hirakata.kmu.ac.jp
7. Department of Pathology, Kansai Medical University, Hirakata 573-1010, Japan; tsutakoj@hirakata.kmu.ac.jp
8. EGID, Inserm, CHU Lille, Institut Pasteur de Lille, U1011, University of Lille, 59019 Lille, France; david.dombrowicz@pasteur-lille.fr
9. Department of Otorhinolaryngology, Shimane University Faculty of Medicine, Izumo 693-0021, Japan; kawauchi@med.shimane-u.ac.jp
10. Department of Otorhinolaryngology Head & Neck Surgery, University of Fukui, Fukui 910-1193, Japan; sfujieda@g.u-fukui.ac.jp
* Correspondence: akanda@hirakata.kmu.ac.jp; Tel.: +81-72-804-0101
† Equally contributed authors.

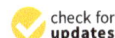

Received: 18 January 2019; Accepted: 30 January 2019; Published: 5 February 2019

Abstract: Background: Chronic rhinosinusitis with nasal polyps (CRSwNP) is a refractory upper airway disease, accompanied mainly by eosinophilia and/or asthma. In addition, the disease correlates with a high rate of hyposmia, following a marked infiltration of eosinophils into the inflamed site, the paranasal sinus. Although eosinophils are known to contribute to the development of hyposmia and CRSwNP pathology, the underlying mechanisms remain unclear. This study aimed to investigate whether eosinophilic upper airway inflammation induces hyposmia and CRSwNP in a murine model using an adoptive transfer system. Methods: To induce eosinophilic rhinosinusitis, splenocytes, including a high proportion (over 50%) of activated eosinophils (SPLhEos), were collected from interleukin-5 transgenic mice following double intraperitoneal injections of antigens, such as ovalbumin, house dust mite, or fungus. Activated SPLhEos with corresponding antigens were then transferred into the nasal cavity of recipient mice, which were sensitized and challenged by the corresponding antigen four times per week. Olfactory function, histopathological, and computed tomography (CT) analyses were performed 2 days after the final transfer of eosinophils. Results: Hyposmia was induced significantly in mice that received SPLhEos transfer compared with healthy and allergic mice, but it did not promote morphological alteration of the paranasal sinus. Pathological analysis revealed that epithelial layer injury and metaplasia similar to polyps, with prominent eosinophil infiltration, was induced in recipient tissue. However, there was no nasal polyp development with interstitial edema that was similar to those recognized in human chronic rhinosinusitis. Conclusions: This study supports the previously unsuspected contribution of eosinophils to CRS development in the murine model and suggests that murine-activated eosinophilic splenocytes contribute to the development of hyposmia due to more mucosal inflammation than physical airway obstruction and epithelial layer injury with convex lesions.

Keywords: allergic rhinitis; chronic rhino sinusitis; nasal poly; eosinophil; hyposmia

1. Introduction

Eosinophils play a critical role in Th2 (T-helper cell type 2)-associated pathology of diseases, such as allergic rhinitis (AR), Th2-skewed chronic rhinosinusitis (CRS), and asthma [1–3]. Eosinophils exert their effect through cytotoxic mediators, comprising granules (eosinophil peroxidase (EPO), major basic protein (MBP), eosinophil cationic protein (ECP), and eosinophil-derived neurotoxin (EDN)), cytokines (Interleukin (IL)-2, IL-4, IL-5, IL-6, IL-10, IL-13, IL-16, IL-18, and transforming growth factor (TGF)-β), chemokines (regulated on activation, normal T cell expressed and secreted (RANTES) and eotaxin), and lipid mediators (platelet-activating factor and leukotriene C4) [1–3]. Eosinophil-derived cytotoxic mediators cause damage to the epithelial layer, airway mucosa, and nerves, resulting subsequently in airway hyperresponsiveness (AHR). Furthermore, profibrotic cytokines and fibrogenic mediators, such as IL-11, IL-17, IL-17E (also known as IL-25), TGF-α, TGFβ1, and matrix metalloproteinase-9, are involved in airway remodeling in asthma [4] and polyp formation in CRS with nasal polyps (CRSwNP) [5]. However, the development of CRSwNP pathogenesis is still poorly understood.

Chronic rhinosinusitis is currently grouped into clinical phenotypes of CRSwNP and CRS without nasal polyps (CRSsNP). Patients with CRSwNP possess a high risk of recurrent sinonasal polyps following endoscopic sinus surgery (ESS) [6], and CRSwNP is closely associated with asthma and characterized by eosinophilia. On the other hand, CRSsNP is generally accompanied by bacterial infection and/or the presence of neutrophils [6]. Regarding mechanisms of CRSwNP development, Bachert et al. previously reported that both orchestration by Th2 cytokines and amplification by *Staphylococcus aureus* enterotoxin B (SEB), a *S. aureus* superantigen, are required for the formation of nasal polyps with eosinophilia [7]. Furthermore, in a recent study of inflammatory endotypes and phenotypes of CRS, CRSwNP, and CRSsNP, based on cluster analysis of biomarkers, Tomassen et al. demonstrated that high expression of IL-5 and the presence of *S. aureus* enterotoxin-specific IgE (SE-IgE) were both observed in patients with CRSwNP, but not in those with CRSsNP [8].

Given that the affected tissue in patients with CRSwNP is frequently infiltrated by large numbers of eosinophils, the name "eosinophilic rhinosinusitis" (ECRS) has been proposed as a new clinically diagnosed phenotype of CRSwNP [9,10]. ECRS is characterized by blood eosinophilia, ethmoid sinus disease detected by computed tomography (CT), bronchial asthma, and aspirin and nonsteroidal anti-inflammatory drug intolerance in CRSwNP [9,10]. Regarding clinical symptoms, the development of hyposmia or anosmia in particular commonly precedes other symptoms, such as nasal obstruction, and is significantly exacerbated in patients with ECRS compared with non-ECRS in CRSwNP [9,10]. Similarly, Klimek et al. previously reported that olfactory dysfunction following specific antigen provocation in patients with grass pollen sensitivity is correlated more closely with the level of inflammatory eosinophil-derived cytotoxic mediators, such as ECP, in nasal secretions than with nasal flow volume measured by active anterior rhinomanometry, suggesting a relationship between olfactory dysfunction and nasal eosinophilic inflammation [11]. Thus, these data indicate that eosinophils directly and/or indirectly cause olfactory damage in inflamed sites. However, no reports exist as to whether eosinophils are capable of directly inducing olfactory dysfunction in ECRS as well as AR.

Understanding the mechanisms behind nasal polyp formation and better informing drug discovery research for ECRS in CRSwNP require not only cluster analyses of human samples but also the development of an animal model of CRSwNP. Concerning the development of CRSwNP in murine models, Kim et al. reported that nasal polypoid lesions could be induced in an AR murine model treated with ovalbumin (OVA) plus SEB [12]. However, studies using this animal disease model have been reported by this one group [12–14].

To assess the essential role of eosinophils in vivo, our group previously reported an eosinophil-derived airway inflammation model via eosinophil transfer into the lower airway of recipient mice through intratracheal administration [15]. In this study, we examined whether splenocytes (containing a large number of eosinophils) transferred into a recipient's nasal cavity can induce CRSwNP with hyposmia.

2. Methods

2.1. Mice

The following mouse strains were used: BALB/c and IL-5 transgenic (Tg) mice (BALB/c background), obtained from Shimizu Laboratory (Kyoto, Japan) and Dr. D. Dombrowicz (Institut Pasteur de Lille, Lille, France), respectively. All mice were housed at 21–23 °C with 40–60% humidity in animal facilities with a 12 h light/dark cycle and were provided food and water ad libitum. All animal experiments were performed using protocols approved by the Kansai Medical University Animal Ethics Committee (18-082).

2.2. Preparation of Splenocytes including a High Number of Activated Eosinophils

To collect activated splenocytes including high proportions of eosinophils (SPLhEos), donor mice (IL-5 Tg) were sensitized with three intraperitoneal injections of PBS or antigen: 50 µg OVA (grade V; Sigma, St. Louis, Missouri, USA), 10 µg *Dermatophagoides farinae* (Der f) house dust mite (HDM) allergen (Institute of Tokyo Environmental Allergy, Tokyo, Japan), or 50 µg *Aspergillus* (Institute of Tokyo Environmental Allergy, Tokyo, Japan) in 2 mg of aluminum hydroxide (Alum) (Thermo Fisher Scientific, Waltham, Massachusetts, USA) on Days 0, 7, and 14 (Figure 1A). Donor mice were sacrificed at Day 15, and splenocytes were prepared. Cells were counted in a hemocytometer and using Diff Quik (Dade Behring AG, Dudingen, Switzerland) following cytospin (Thermo Shandon, Pittsburgh, PA, USA). The eosinophil percentage among splenocytes was greater than 50%. The character of splenocytes from IL-5 Tg mouse as determined by flow cytometric analysis is shown in Figure S1.

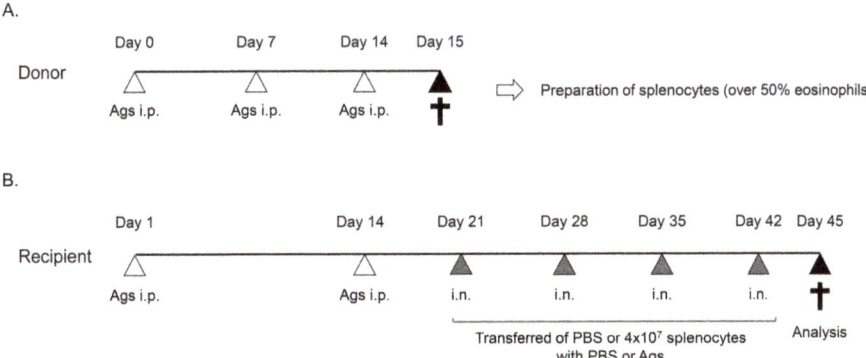

Figure 1. Experimental design of the adoptive transfer system. (**A**). Preparation of activated splenocytes from the donor. Donor IL-5 Tg mice were sensitized with three intraperitoneal (i.p.) injections of antigens (Ags): ovalbumin (OVA), *Dermatophagoides farinae* (Der f), or *Aspergillus*. Splenocytes including a high number of eosinophils (SPLhEos) were collected from spleens of IL-5 Tg mice 24 h after the final injection.

(**B**) Protocol for adoptive transfer into recipient mice. After recipient mice had been sensitized with (i.p.) injections of corresponding Ags for the donor, 4×10^7 splenocytes were transferred into the nasal cavity of recipient mice via intranasal (i.n.) injections. "Control animals" indicates transfer of PBS or SPLhEos with phosphate buffered saline (PBS). Simultaneously, PBS or corresponding Ags were also administrated alongside SPLhEos via i.n. injections.

2.3. Adoptive Transfer System

To induce activated ECRS in a murine model, an eosinophil adoptive transfer system was designed, as shown in Figure 1B [15,16]. Recipient mice were sensitized with PBS or corresponding antigens on Days 0 and 14. Following splenocyte preparation, 2×10^6 activated SPLhEos in 30 µL phosphate-buffered saline (PBS) alone, PBS with 0.5% OVA, 1 µg Der f, or 10 µg *Aspergillus* (or the same allergens alone in PBS, or PBS alone) were transferred into the nasal cavity of recipients sensitized with PBS or corresponding antigens by intranasal administration into both nostrils, once per week (4 times at each instance) for 4 weeks, on Days 21, 28, 35, and 42. Administration was performed under systemic anesthesia with 0.5 mg/kg medetomidine (Domitor; Pfizer, New York, NY, USA) and 50 mg/kg ketamine (Ketalar; Daiichi-Sankyo, Tokyo, Japan). In HDM- and *Aspergillus*-sensitized mice, 1 mg/µL SEB (Sigma) or 2 µM DNA containing unmethylated CpG motifs (CpGDNA: ODN2395; type B; Cosmo Bio, Tokyo, Japan) was also administered along with SPLhEos. Recipient mice were then evaluated via a functional assay (buried food test), histological analysis, and CT analysis at 48 h post the final SPLhEos transfer.

2.4. Buried Food Test

Buried food tests to evaluate the olfactory function of mice were performed 48 h after the final SPLhEos according to Yang et al.'s method, with some modifications [17]. Food deprivation was initiated 24 h prior to the test by removing pellets from the food hopper of the home cage. During the test, a clean cage was prepared (44 cm L × 29.2 cm W × 20 cm H) containing a 3 cm depth of clean bedding. The subject mouse was transferred to the test cage, allowed to acclimatize for 5 min, and then returned to the original cage. After the mouse had been returned to the home cage, one piece of cookie (Tabekko Dobutsu Biscuits, Ginbisu, Tokyo, Japan) was buried in a random corner, approximately 1 cm beneath the surface of the test cage. The subject mouse was then transferred to the middle of the test cage and latency was measured between the time point of transfer and the subject mouse finding the buried food. If the subject had failed to find the buried food after 5 min had elapsed, the test was stopped and 300 s was recorded as the latency score.

2.5. Histological Analysis

To prepare paraffin sections 48 h after the final transfer of SPLhEos, recipient mice were fixed through cardiac perfusion with 10% neutral buffered formalin (Muto Kagaku, Tokyo, Japan) under deep anesthesia and decapitated. Trimmed heads, including nasal cavity, were then locally irrigated using the same fixative at room temperature for 1 week, followed by decalcification in 10% ethylenediaminetetraacetic acid (pH 7.0) at room temperature for 2 weeks. Following decalcification, coronal sections (4 µm thick) on the level of the anterior end of the olfactory bulb were mounted on Matsunami-adhesive-silane (MAS)-coated slides (Matsunami Glass, Osaka, Japan). For human samples, the use of nasal polyps from patients with CRSwNP was approved by the local ethics committee of University of Tokyo Hospital (12009).

To prepare frozen sections, following decapitation, trimmed heads were immediately frozen in isopentane (nacalai tesque, Kyoto, Japan) cooled in liquid nitrogen, then freeze-embedded with super cryoembedding medium (SCEM, Leica Microsystems, Land Hessen, Germany) in coolant. Fresh frozen samples were sectioned using a film method without fixation or decalcification (the "unfixed and undecalcified method"), known as the Kawamoto method [18]. Fresh-frozen sections (4 µm thick) were mounted on Cryofilm (Leica Microsystems).

Sections were stained with hematoxylin and eosin (H&E) for morphological analysis or Sirius red staining for visualization of eosinophils. Histological analyses were assessed by two different pathologists.

2.6. Computed tomography Analysis

Computed tomography scans were performed immediately on mice sacrificed 48 h after the last transfer, using a Siemens Inveon Micro-CT (Siemens, Bayern, Germany). Images were calibrated for Hounsfield unit scaling using a water-filled phantom on each experiment day. The scanner settings were as follows: tube voltage of 70 kVp and current of 500 µA over 360 continuous projections with an exposure time of 1000 ms per projection. Cross-sectional images were reconstructed using Inveon Viewer Quick Launch (Siemens) and converted to the Digital Imaging and Communications in Medicine (DICOM) format using PMOD software (PMOD Technologies LLC, Zurich, Switzerland).

2.7. Statistical Analysis

Data are presented as means ± standard errors of the mean (SEMs). Statistical significance was determined using the Mann–Whitney U test in the buried food test. The threshold of significance was set at $p < 0.05$ for all tests.

A Supplementary Materials section can be found in the online repository for this article.

3. Results

3.1. Hyposmia on Transfer of SPLhEos in Th2-Skewed Response

To investigate the functional role of Th-2 skewed SPLhEos in vivo, an adoptive transfer system was performed with Th2 polarization. SPLhEos activated by OVA were transferred into OVA-sensitized recipients; the buried food test was then performed to assess olfactory dysfunction, followed by histological analysis. As shown in Figure 2A, the olfactory dysfunction assay revealed that hyposmia was significantly induced on adoptive transfer of SPLhEos with OVA in recipient mice (118 ± 48.8 s) compared with OVA alone (27.6 ± 8.9 s) ($p = 0.047$). However, there were no clear differences in morphological change of the paranasal sinus (in paraffin sections) between groups, or in the development of nasal polypoid lesions (Figure 2B).

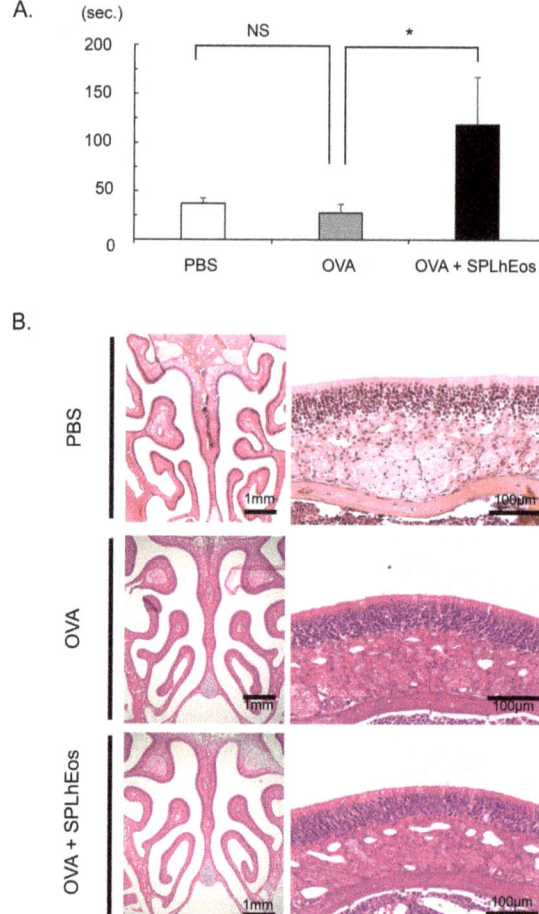

Figure 2. Buried food test (**A**) and histological analysis (**B**) following the transfer of SPLhEos in Th2-skewed response. (**A**.) Open, gray, and black bars indicate the transfer of PBS alone, OVA alone, and OVA + SPLhEos (4×10^7 cells) in the adoptive transfer system, respectively. Data are expressed as means ± SEM of $n = 5$ mice per group. * Statistically significant difference from control mice ($p < 0.05$). (**B**) Hematoxylin and eosin (H&E) staining of histological sections.

3.2. Epithelia Injury on Transfer of SPLhEos in Adoptive and Innate Responses

As HDMs promote eosinophilic airway inflammation with AHR (Figure S2A) and are implicated in both adaptive and innate immune responses [19,20], donor and recipient mice were sensitized with HDM, and adoptive transfers were performed with HDM. As shown in Figure 3A, upon transfer of SPLhEos activated by HDM and HDM, convex lesions were observed in the epithelial layer of the paranasal sinus with no evidence of nasal polyps present in humans being observed in the paraffin sections of mice also treated with SEB, which modulates innate immunity. Upon transfer of SPLhEos activated by HDM with HDM plus SEB, a more pronounced epithelial injury was observed in paraffin sections. Histological analyses of frozen sections using the unfixed and undecalcified method (reflecting near-physiological morphology) revealed no clear differences in physiological morphology among these groups. Furthermore, swelling of the nasal mucosa was barely observed in any of the groups. Similar results were observed in the CT analysis (Figure 3B).

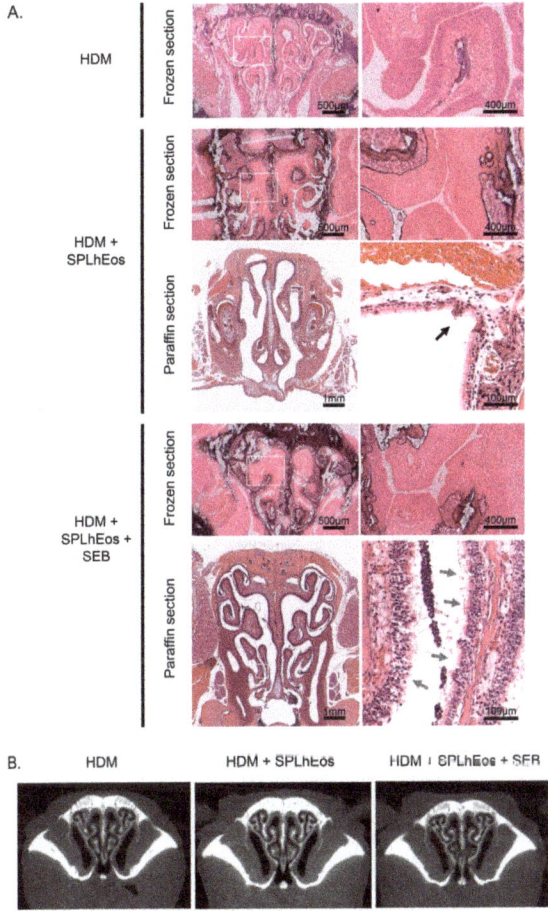

Figure 3. Histological (**A**) and CT (**B**) analyses on the transfer of SPLhEos with house dust mite (HDM). Transfer of HDM alone, HDM with SPLhEos (4×10^7 cells), and HDM with SPLhEos (4×10^7 cells) plus *Staphylococcus aureus* enterotoxin B (SEB) were grouped into the adoptive transfer system (two individual experiments with $n = 4$ or 5 mice per group). Subfigures (**A**,**B**) indicate histology in H&E-stained frozen and paraffin-embedded sections, and coronal images taken by the CT scan in the paranasal sinus, respectively.

Allergic fungal rhinosinusitis, such as *Aspergillus* infection, is an additional subtype in CRSwNP, with the fungus not only promoting eosinophilic airway inflammation with AHR (Figure S2B) similar to OVA and HDM, but also inducing toll-like receptor (TLR) expression [21–23]. Therefore, to investigate whether *Aspergillus* induces upper airway inflammation similar to ECRS, adoptive *Aspergillus* with/without SPLhEos was transferred into *Aspergillus*-sensitized recipient mice. As shown in Figure 4, on transfer of *Aspergillus* with SPLhEos, severe epithelial layer injury, numerous convex lesions, and marked eosinophilic infiltration into the mucosal layer were observed compared with *Aspergillus* alone; however, no nasal polyps like in humans were found. To induce a more powerful immune response, SEB or CpGDNA were administered alongside SPLhEos and *Aspergillus* as TLR9 agonists. However, no clear histological differences were observed among SPLhEos with *Aspergillus*, with *Aspergillus* plus SEB, or with *Aspergillus* plus CpGDNA. In micro-CT analysis, nasal polyps, observed in ECRS, were observed in none of the groups. Thus, treatment with SEB or CpGDNA exerted no amplification effects.

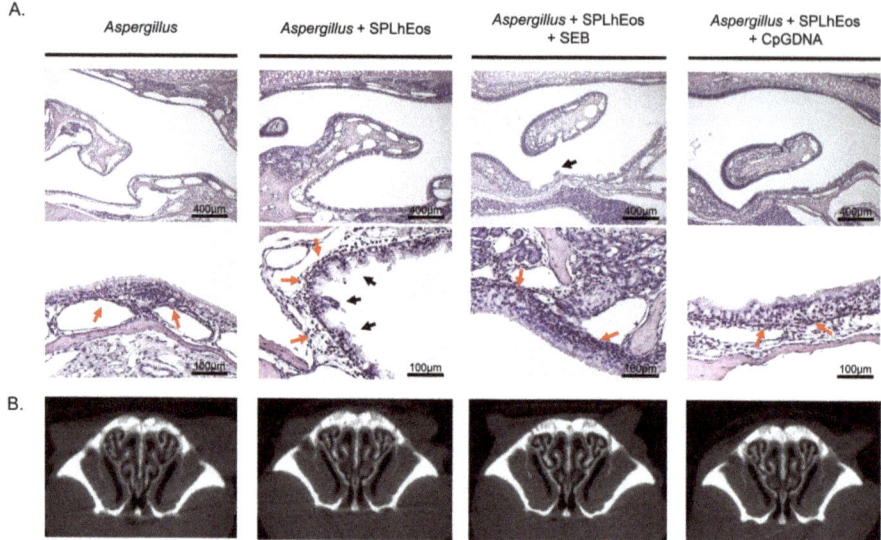

Figure 4. Histological (**A**) and CT (**B**) analyses on the transfer of SPLhEos with *Aspergillus*. Transfer of *Aspergillus* alone, *Aspergillus* with SPLhEos (4 × 10^7 cells), *Aspergillus* with SPLhEos (4 × 10^7 cells) plus *Staphylococcus aureus* enterotoxin B (SEB), or *Aspergillus* with SPLhEos (4 × 10^7 cells) plus DNA containing unmethylated CpG motifs (CpGDNA) were grouped into the adoptive transfer system (n = 5 mice per group). Subfigures (**A**,**B**) indicate Sirius-red-stained histological sections and coronal images taken by CT scans in the paranasal sinus, respectively.

3.3. Thin Tissue Component of Turbinate in Murine Paranasal Sinuses

Histological differences between human and murine paranasal sinuses are shown in Figure 5. In humans, the turbinate comprises a rich stromal component with serous glands, while the maxillary sinus comprises poor submucosal tissue (Figure 5A). In contrast, the murine tissue composition is the inverse of that in human (Figure 5B); characteristics of histological differences of the paranasal sinus between humans and mice are summarized in Table 1. From histological findings in CRSwNP following ESS, nasal polyps commonly consist of a thin epithelial layer with prominent edema and marked proinflammatory cells (mainly eosinophils) (Figure 5C). However, the nasal polypoid lesions in Figures 3 and 4 seem to comprise epithelial metaplasias with injury of the epithelial layer, rather than nasal polyps in ECRS.

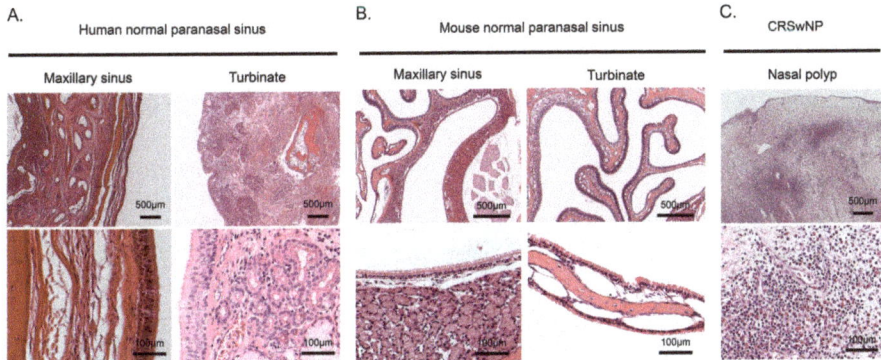

Figure 5. Histology of normal human paranasal sinus (**A**), normal mouse paranasal sinus (**B**), and nasal polyps from chronic rhinosinusitis with nasal polyps (CRSwNP) (**C**). Histological sections were stained using H&E.

Table 1. Characteristics of human and mouse paranasal sinuses.

	Maxillary Sinus			Turbinate		
	Mucosal Layer	Interstitium Tissue	Gland	Mucosal Layer	Interstitium Tissue	Gland
Human	Thin	Poor	Poor	Thick	Rich	Rich
Mouse	Thin–moderate	Poor	Rich	Thin	Poor	Poor

4. Discussion

We aimed to investigate whether eosinophilia during upper airway inflammation induces olfactory disturbance and/or promotes nasal polyp formation in the CRS using an adoptive transfer system with activated SPLhEos. Our results demonstrate that SPLhEos-induced upper airway inflammation results in hyposmia, but morphological alteration of the paranasal sinus was not promoted. This paper is the first to report a direct contribution of eosinophilic upper airway inflammation in olfactory disturbance. Olfactory disturbance is a common symptom of CRSwNP [24], especially as an initial symptom of ECRS [10]. There are two possible mechanisms of olfactory disturbance: (1) closing of the olfactory cleft, which occurs during nasal septum obstruction by nasal polyps, or (2) olfactory neuroepithelium injury following mucosal inflammation [25,26]. Doty et al. reported that there was little correlation between airway patency and olfactory function, except in the case of complete or almost complete blockage of the olfactory cleft, resulting in odorant molecules not gaining access to the olfactory mucosa [27]. Thus, this report suggests that hyposmia in our model is due to mucosal inflammation rather than physical airway obstruction. Our observations of hyposmia without morphological changes or nasal obstruction of the olfactory cleft suggest that hyposmia may be induced by eosinophil-derived toxic mediators following olfactory neuroepithelium injury. This is suggested as eosinophil-derived granules have a capability of inducing tissue damage and dysfunction [1,28]. Causes of hyposmia require further investigation for treatment of patients with ECRS, as no studies have been reported on direct injury of the neuroepithelium by eosinophil-derived mediators.

CRSwNP including ECRS is a heterogeneous disease that is identified by various inflammatory endotypes [8,29,30]; its pathogenesis implicates three major types of innate and adaptive cell-mediated effector immunity: type 1 (natural killer cells, innate lymphoid cell (ILC)1, cytotoxic T (Tc)1, and Th1), type 2 (ILC2, Tc2, and Th2), and type 3 (ILC3, Tc17, and Th17) immune responses [30,31]. Recent reports have suggested that increased expression of TLRs (TLR2, 4, 7, and 9) and protease-activated receptors contributes to the development of CRS [5,32,33]. Furthermore, the expressions of TLR1–7, 9, and 10 have been identified in eosinophils, a key player in CRSwNP [1]. Notably, it has been reported that SEB not only enhances Th2 response through interaction with TLR2 signaling [34,35] but also plays a potential role in IL-5, IL-13, and RANTES production in dispersed nasal polyps following the development of CRSwNP [36]. Supporting this, high concentrations of *S. aureus* enterotoxin-specific IgE are associated with nasal polyps with intense eosinophilic inflammation [8]. Regarding molecular pathogenesis, HDM induces both adaptive and innate immune responses through protease-activated receptor (PAR) 2 via proteases [37], and TLR2 and 4 [19,20], whereas OVA contributes only to antigen-specific reactions, reflecting Th2-adaptive immune responses. Similarly, *Aspergillus* induces the signaling of TLRs (TLR1, 2, 3, 4, 6, and 9) [21–23] in a wider range than HDM. Therefore, we also investigated the effects of HDM and *Aspergillus* in the adoptive SPLhEos transfer system. However, no nasal polyps were observed like those seen in patients with CRSwNP, although more severe damage of the epithelial layer was observed following the development of convex lesions.

Moreover, we assess SPLhEos-induced upper airway inflammation because micro-CT analysis can be used to detect the physiological and pathological morphology of the paranasal sinus. Although micro-CT analysis was confirmed as a useful method to detect the swelling of the nasal mucosa following the methacholine challenge test (Figure S3), no morphological changes were observed in this experimental model. Thus, these results indicate that eosinophilic upper airway inflammation in a murine model using an adoptive transfer system does not induce mucosal irregularity with edema like those seen in CT images of patients with CRSwNP.

Regarding a CRSwNP animal model, Kim et al. reported an animal model of CRSwNP through frequent nasal instillation of SEB, CpGDNA, or *Aspergillus* protease under OVA-induced, Th2-skewed immune response, which required >100 days for the development of nasal polyps [12–14]. They found not only nasal polyps or polypoid lesions with epithelial thickening and infiltration of inflammatory cells, but also mucosal irregularity of nasal polyps by micro-CT analysis [12–14]. We observed convex lesions (polypoid lesion) with hallmark eosinophil infiltration, similar to the findings by Kim et al. However, two different pathologists indicated that these nasal polypoid lesions are similar to reactive granuloma with epithelial hyperplasia, and not the same as nasal polyps in humans. This is because polyps usually consist of edematous mucosa with a loose stroma and a variety of inflammatory cell infiltration (seen in Figure 5C). In this pathological change, a small widened stroma was observed, filled with small/capillary vessels and inflammatory cells, with no edema. Furthermore, as summarized in Table 1, histological structures are completely different between humans and mice. Thus, in a murine model, these findings suggest that it could be experimentally difficult to induce the development of nasal polyps like in humans.

In conclusion, we report that eosinophilic upper airway inflammation induces hyposmia using an adoptive transfer system into the nasal cavity. Analysis of hyposmia using the adoptive SPLhEos transfer model may be a useful examination method for understanding disease mechanisms or developing new drugs for olfactory disorders. Regarding the CRSwNP murine model, our data and previous reports suggest that additional studies are essential, but that caution is required in future investigations when using these models.

Supplementary Materials: The following are available online at http://www.mdpi.com/2076-3271/7/2/22/s1. Figure S1: Flow cytometric analysis of splenocytes from IL-5 transgenic mouse, Figure S2: Induction of allergic airway inflammation by HDM (A) and Aspergillus (B), Figure S3: CT analysis images in the paranasal sinus. Left and right panels indicate coronal sections in control (PBS/PBS) and OVA-sensitized and challenged groups (OVA/OVA), respectively; and online supplementary methods.

Author Contributions: A.K. and K.K. were involved in all stages of this investigation. Y.K., B.D., K.S., S.S., Y.S. and B.B. performed the experiments. N.H. and K.T. commented on the pathological findings. M.A., A.N., K.T., D.D., H.K., S.F. and H.I. were involved in technical comments and drafting the manuscript. All authors approved the final manuscript and publication.

Funding: This work was supported by funding from the Academic Society for Research in Otolaryngology, Kansai Medical University; a research grant from Kansai Medical University (KMU) research consortium; the Ministry of Education, Culture, Sports, Science and Technology (MEXT)-Supported Program for the Strategic Research Foundation at Private Universities (S1201038); a Grant-in-Aid for Scientific Research (C) from MEXT (15K10793); and Grants-in-Aid for Scientific Research from the Japanese Ministry of Health, Labor and Welfare (H26-, H27-Research on measures for intractable disease-general-004).

Acknowledgments: We thank Yumiko Kouno, Keita Utsunomiya, and Tanigawa Noboru (Department of Radiology, Kansai Medical University) for their technical advice and assistance. The authors would like to thank Enago (www.enago.jp) for the English language review.

Conflicts of Interest: The authors declare no conflict of interest. The founding sponsors had no role in the design of the study.

Abbreviations

AR, allergic rhinitis; Alum, aluminum hydroxide; CRS, chronic rhinosinusitis; CRSwNP, chronic rhinosinusitis with nasal polyp; CRSsNP, chronic rhinosinusitis without nasal polyp; CT, computer tomography; ECP, eosinophil cationic protein; ESS, endoscopic sinus surgery; ECRS, eosinophilic chronic rhinosinusitis; EDN, eosinophil-derived neurotoxin; EPO, eosinophil peroxidase; Der f, *Dermatophagoides farinae*; HDM, house dust mite; i.n., intranasal; i.p., intraperitoneal; i.t., intratracheal; JESREC, Japanese Epidemiological Survey of Refractory Eosinophilic Chronic Rhinosinusitis; ILC, innate lymphoid cell; IL, interleukin; MBP, major basic protein; MCH, methacholine; MMP, matrix metalloproteinase; NK, natural killer; OVA, ovalbumin; PAR, protease-activated receptor; SAE, *Staphylococcus aureus* enterotoxin; SAgs, superantigens; SEA, staphylococcal enterotoxin A; SEB, *Staphylococcus aureus* enterotoxin B; SE-IgE, *Staphylococcus aureus* enterotoxin-specific IgE; SPLhEos, splenocytes including a high number of eosinophils; Tc, cytotoxic T; TGF, transforming growth factor; Tg, transgenic; Th, T helper cell type; TLR, toll-like receptor.

References

1. Rothenberg, M.E.; Hogan, S.P. The eosinophil. *Annu. Rev. Immunol.* **2006**, *24*, 147–174. [CrossRef] [PubMed]
2. Blanchard, C.; Rothenberg, M.E. Biology of the eosinophil. *Adv. Immunol.* **2009**, *101*, 81–121. [CrossRef] [PubMed]
3. Rosenberg, H.F.; Dyer, K.D.; Foster, P.S. Eosinophils: Changing perspectives in health and disease. *Nat. Rev. Immunol.* **2013**, *13*, 9–22. [CrossRef] [PubMed]
4. Foley, S.C.; Prefontaine, D.; Hamid, Q. Images in allergy and immunology: Role of eosinophils in airway remodeling. *J. Allergy Clin. Immunol.* **2007**, *119*, 1563–1566. [CrossRef]
5. Schleimer, R.P. Immunopathogenesis of Chronic Rhinosinusitis and Nasal Polyposis. *Annu. Rev. Pathol.* **2017**, *12*, 331–357. [CrossRef] [PubMed]
6. Fokkens, W.J.; Lund, V.J.; Mullol, J.; Bachert, C.; Alobid, I.; Baroody, F.; Cohen, N.; Cervin, A.; Douglas, R.; Gevaert, P.; et al. European Position Paper on Rhinosinusitis and Nasal Polyps. *Rhinol. Suppl.* **2012**, *23*, 1–298.
7. Bachert, C.; Zhang, N.; Holtappels, G.; De Lobel, L.; van Cauwenberge, P.; Liu, S.; Lin, P.; Bousquet, J.; Van Steen, K. Presence of IL-5 protein and IgE antibodies to staphylococcal enterotoxins in nasal polyps is associated with comorbid asthma. *J. Allergy Clin. Immunol.* **2010**, *126*, 962–968.e6. [CrossRef]
8. Tomassen, P.; Vandeplas, G.; Van Zele, T.; Cardell, L.O.; Arebro, J.; Olze, H.; Forster-Ruhrmann, U.; Kowalski, M.L.; Olszewska-Ziaber, A.; Holtappels, G.; et al. Inflammatory endotypes of chronic rhinosinusitis based on cluster analysis of biomarkers. *J. Allergy Clin. Immunol.* **2016**, *137*, 1449–1456.e4. [CrossRef]
9. Sakuma, Y.; Ishitoya, J.; Komatsu, M.; Shiono, O.; Hirama, M.; Yamashita, Y.; Kaneko, T.; Morita, S.; Tsukuda, M. New clinical diagnostic criteria for eosinophilic chronic rhinosinusitis. *Auris Nasus Larynx* **2011**, *38*, 583–588. [CrossRef]
10. Tokunaga, T.; Sakashita, M.; Haruna, T.; Asaka, D.; Takeno, S.; Ikeda, H.; Nakayama, T.; Seki, N.; Ito, S.; Murata, J.; et al. Novel scoring system and algorithm for classifying chronic rhinosinusitis: The JESREC Study. *Allergy* **2015**, *70*, 995–1003. [CrossRef]
11. Klimek, L.; Eggers, G. Olfactory dysfunction in allergic rhinitis is related to nasal eosinophilic inflammation. *J. Allergy Clin. Immunol.* **1997**, *100*, 158–164. [CrossRef]
12. Kim, D.W.; Khalmuratova, R.; Hur, D.G.; Jeon, S.Y.; Kim, S.W.; Shin, H.W.; Lee, C.H.; Rhee, C.S. *Staphylococcus aureus* enterotoxin B contributes to induction of nasal polypoid lesions in an allergic rhinosinusitis murine model. *Am. J. Rhinol. Allergy* **2011**, *25*, e255–e261. [CrossRef] [PubMed]
13. Kim, S.W.; Kim, D.W.; Khalmuratova, R.; Kim, J.H.; Jung, M.H.; Chang, D.Y.; Shin, E.C.; Lee, H.K.; Shin, H.W.; Rhee, C.S.; et al. Resveratrol prevents development of eosinophilic rhinosinusitis with nasal polyps in a mouse model. *Allergy* **2013**, *68*, 862–869. [CrossRef] [PubMed]
14. Kim, H.C.; Lim, J.Y.; Kim, S.; Kim, J.H.; Jang, Y.J. Development of a mouse model of eosinophilic chronic rhinosinusitis with nasal polyp by nasal instillation of an *Aspergillus* protease and ovalbumin. *Eur. Arch. Oto-Rhino-Laryngol.* **2017**, *274*, 3899–3906. [CrossRef] [PubMed]

15. Kanda, A.; Driss, V.; Hornez, N.; Abdallah, M.; Roumier, T.; Abboud, G.; Legrand, F.; Staumont-Salle, D.; Queant, S.; Bertout, J.; et al. Eosinophil-derived IFN-gamma induces airway hyperresponsiveness and lung inflammation in the absence of lymphocytes. *J. Allergy Clin. Immunol.* **2009**, *124*, 573–582. [CrossRef] [PubMed]
16. Wen, T.; Besse, J.A.; Mingler, M.K.; Fulkerson, P.C.; Rothenberg, M.E. Eosinophil adoptive transfer system to directly evaluate pulmonary eosinophil trafficking in vivo. *Proc. Natl. Acad. Sci. USA* **2013**, *110*, 6067–6072. [CrossRef] [PubMed]
17. Yang, M.; Crawley, J.N. Simple behavioral assessment of mouse olfaction. *Curr. Protoc. Neurosci.* **2009**, *8*, 8–24. [CrossRef]
18. Kawamoto, T. Use of a new adhesive film for the preparation of multi-purpose fresh-frozen sections from hard tissues, whole-animals, insects and plants. *Arch. Histol. Cytol.* **2003**, *66*, 123–143. [CrossRef]
19. Ryu, J.H.; Yoo, J.Y.; Kim, M.J.; Hwang, S.G.; Ahn, K.C.; Ryu, J.C.; Choi, M.K.; Joo, J.H.; Kim, C.H.; Lee, S.N.; et al. Distinct TLR-mediated pathways regulate house dust mite-induced allergic disease in the upper and lower airways. *J. Allergy Clin. Immunol.* **2013**, *131*, 549–561. [CrossRef]
20. Liu, C.F.; Drocourt, D.; Puzo, G.; Wang, J.Y.; Riviere, M. Innate immune response of alveolar macrophage to house dust mite allergen is mediated through TLR2/-4 co-activation. *PLoS ONE* **2013**, *8*, e75983. [CrossRef]
21. Schubert, M.S. Allergic fungal sinusitis: Pathophysiology, diagnosis and management. *Med. Mycol.* **2009**, *47*, S324–S330. [CrossRef] [PubMed]
22. Chakrabarti, A.; Kaur, H. Allergic Aspergillus Rhinosinusitis. *J. Fungi* **2016**, *2*. [CrossRef] [PubMed]
23. Williams, P.B.; Barnes, C.S.; Portnoy, J.M. Innate and Adaptive Immune Response to Fungal Products and Allergens. *J. Allergy Clin. Immunol. Pract.* **2016**, *4*, 386–395. [CrossRef] [PubMed]
24. Stevens, W.W.; Schleimer, R.P.; Kern, R.C. Chronic Rhinosinusitis with Nasal Polyps. *J. Allergy Clin. Immunol. Pract.* **2016**, *4*, 565–572. [CrossRef] [PubMed]
25. Gaines, A.D. Anosmia and hyposmia. *Allergy Asthma Proc.* **2010**, *31*, 185–189. [CrossRef] [PubMed]
26. Syed, I.; Philpott, C. Hyposmia. *Br. J. Hosp. Med.* **2015**, *76*, C41–C42. [CrossRef] [PubMed]
27. Doty, R.L. Office procedures for quantitative assessment of olfactory function. *Am. J. Rhinol.* **2007**, *21*, 460–473. [CrossRef]
28. Yang, D.; Chen, Q.; Su, S.B.; Zhang, P.; Kurosaka, K.; Caspi, R.R.; Michalek, S.M.; Rosenberg, H.F.; Zhang, N.; Oppenheim, J.J. Eosinophil-derived neurotoxin acts as an alarmin to activate the TLR2-MyD88 signal pathway in dendritic cells and enhances Th2 immune responses. *J. Exp. Med.* **2008**, *205*, 79–90. [CrossRef]
29. Li, X.; Hawkins, G.A.; Ampleford, E.J.; Moore, W.C.; Li, H.; Hastie, A.T.; Howard, T.D.; Boushey, H.A.; Busse, W.W.; Calhoun, W.J.; et al. Genome-wide association study identifies TH1 pathway genes associated with lung function in asthmatic patients. *J. Allergy Clin. Immunol.* **2013**, *132*, 313–320. [CrossRef]
30. Cao, P.P.; Wang, Z.C.; Schleimer, R.P.; Liu, Z. Pathophysiologic mechanisms of chronic rhinosinusitis and their roles in emerging disease endotypes. *Ann. Allergy Asthma Immunol.* **2018**. [CrossRef]
31. Annunziato, F.; Romagnani, C.; Romagnani, S. The 3 major types of innate and adaptive cell-mediated effector immunity. *J. Allergy Clin. Immunol.* **2015**, *135*, 626–635. [CrossRef]
32. Zhang, Q.; Wang, C.S.; Han, D.M.; Sy, C.; Huang, Q.; Sun, Y.; Fan, E.Z.; Li, Y.; Zhou, B. Differential expression of Toll-like receptor pathway genes in chronic rhinosinusitis with or without nasal polyps. *Acta Oto-Laryngol.* **2013**, *133*, 165–173. [CrossRef] [PubMed]
33. Park, S.K.; Jin, S.Y.; Yeon, S.H.; Lee, S.B.; Xu, J.; Yoon, Y.H.; Rha, K.S.; Kim, Y.M. Role of Toll-like receptor 9 signaling on activation of nasal polyp-derived fibroblasts and its association with nasal polypogenesis. *Int. Forum Allergy Rhinol.* **2018**, *8*, 1001–1012. [CrossRef] [PubMed]
34. Mandron, M.; Aries, M.F.; Brehm, R.D.; Tranter, H.S.; Acharya, K.R.; Charveron, M.; Davrinche, C. Human dendritic cells conditioned with Staphylococcus aureus enterotoxin B promote TH2 cell polarization. *J. Allergy Clin. Immunol.* **2006**, *117*, 1141–1147. [CrossRef] [PubMed]
35. Forbes-Blom, E.; Camberis, M.; Prout, M.; Tang, S.C.; Le Gros, G. Staphylococcal-derived superantigen enhances peanut induced Th2 responses in the skin. *Clin. Exp. Allergy J. Br. Soc. Allergy Clin. Immunol.* **2012**, *42*, 305–314. [CrossRef]

36. Okano, M.; Fujiwara, T.; Haruna, T.; Kariya, S.; Makihara, S.; Higaki, T.; Nishizaki, K. Role of fungal antigens in eosinophilia-associated cellular responses in nasal polyps: A comparison with enterotoxin. *Clin. Exp. Allergy J. Br. Soc. Allergy Clin. Immunol.* **2011**, *41*, 171–178. [CrossRef] [PubMed]
37. Davidson, C.E.; Asaduzzaman, M.; Arizmendi, N.G.; Polley, D.; Wu, Y.; Gordon, J.R.; Hollenberg, M.D.; Cameron, L.; Vliagoftis, H. Proteinase-activated receptor-2 activation participates in allergic sensitization to house dust mite allergens in a murine model. *Clin. Exp. Allergy* **2013**, *43*, 1274–1285. [CrossRef]

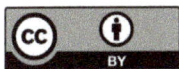

© 2019 by the authors. Licensee MDPI, Basel, Switzerland. This article is an open access article distributed under the terms and conditions of the Creative Commons Attribution (CC BY) license (http://creativecommons.org/licenses/by/4.0/).

MDPI
St. Alban-Anlage 66
4052 Basel
Switzerland
Tel. +41 61 683 77 34
Fax +41 61 302 89 18
www.mdpi.com

Medical Sciences Editorial Office
E-mail: medsci@mdpi.com
www.mdpi.com/journal/medsci